CONTENTS

FOREWORD

Knowledge related to infant hearing, newborn hearing screening, and diagnostic assessment of auditory function in infants continues to advance in numerous directions. The impetus for, and subsequent success of, programs of early detection of hearing loss and intervention were built on a solid foundation that demonstrated the value of early detection of hearing loss and the importance of early intervention in facilitating language development. This success has been facilitated by the availability of proven technology that allows accurate assessment of hearing in the newborn period. Subsequent accumulation of outcomes data and measures of the effectiveness of early intervention underscore the value and facilitate implementation of newborn hearing programs around the world.

With successes come new challenges. As aspects of development of the human auditory system have been characterized, much effort has focused on embryology, whereas developmental changes that occur after birth have not been examined as extensively. Excellent research has focused on cochlear and brainstem function and provided important information about factors that influence otoacoustic emission (OAE) and auditory brainstem response (ABR) measures at various ages. In contrast, less attention has been paid to changes in middle ear function in normal infants, how changes over time may affect outcomes of OAE and ABR tests, and how such characteristics are affected by pathology. A thorough understanding of middle ear function and characteristics in this population is needed, due to the intricate involvement of the middle ear system in the sound transmission pathway. Infant middle ears undergo changes during early life that in turn affect characteristics of responses within and beyond the middle ear system. The importance of such factors is demonstrated by the generally accepted use of higher-frequency probe tones and the expanding interest in wideband reflectance in infant evaluation. Sensitive approaches are likely to advance understanding of normal and abnormal function and contribute to improve test accuracy. All of these topics are addressed in this text.

Middle ear measures and influences on middle ear function involve neural pathways as well. Neural pathways through the brainstem show maturation over the first year of life, as has long been demonstrated by changes in the ABR. Another measure sensitive to eighth nerve/brainstem function is the middle ear muscle reflex (MEMR), a commonly used clinical measure in children and adults but often ignored in infants. In combination with OAEs, MEMRs can provide a method of screening for neural pathway abnormalities, such as auditory neuropathy/dyssynchrony and a valuable diagnostic crosscheck. Appropriate clinical implementation in infants will come with enhanced understanding of the developmental features of the MEMR pathway.

The material contained within this text is contemporary, clinically relevant, and important. Drs. Kei and Zhao and the authors they have brought together for this text provide thoughtful treatises on the current state of our understanding of middle ear function in infants and address needs for refining the accuracy of hearing screening and diagnostic methods utilized with infants. Their careful reviews and thoughtful insights will contribute to continued advancement in meeting the challenges presented by our youngest listeners.

Linda J. Hood, PhD
Professor, Vanderbilt University
Honorary Professor, University
   of Queensland
July 2011

Middle Eas

This book is due for return not later than the last date stamped below, unless recalled sooner.

Assessing Middle Ear Function in Infants

Edited by

JOSEPH KEI, PhD, MAudSA, CCP
Associate Professor
Head—Division of Audiology
Hearing Research Unit for Children
School of Health and Rehabilitation Sciences
University of Queensland
Queensland, Australia

and

FEI ZHAO, MD, PhD
Senior Lecturer
Director—Centre for Hearing and Balance Studies
University of Bristol
Bristol, United Kingdom

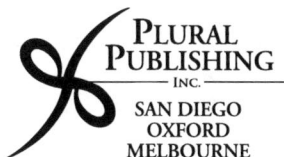

PLURAL
PUBLISHING
INC.
SAN DIEGO
OXFORD
MELBOURNE

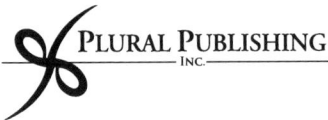

PLURAL PUBLISHING
INC.

5521 Ruffin Road
San Diego, CA 92123

e-mail: info@pluralpublishing.com
Web site: http://www.pluralpublishing.com

49 Bath Street
Abingdon, Oxfordshire OX14 1EA
United Kingdom

Typeset in 11/14 Garamond by Flanagan's Publishing Services, Inc.
Printed in the United States of America by McNaughton & Gunn.

Library of Congress Cataloging-in-Publication Data

Assessing middle ear function in infants / [edited by] Joseph Kei and Fei Zhao.
  p. ; cm.
Includes bibliographical references and index.
ISBN-13: 978-1-59756-391-8 (alk. paper)
ISBN-10: 1-59756-391-9 (alk. paper)
I. Kei, Joseph, 1953- II. Zhao, Fei, 1965-
[DNLM: 1. Acoustic Impedance Tests. 2. Ear, Middle—physiology. 3. Infant. WV 272]
LC classification not assigned
617.8'4—dc23
        2011034085

PREFACE

For the past two decades, significant improvement in the early identification and habilitation of childhood hearing loss has occurred, following the rapid development and widespread implementation of universal newborn hearing screening programs around the world. Many advanced technologies have been developed and implemented to facilitate accurate diagnosis and appropriate management in children with hearing impairment. These include otoacoustic emissions, frequency-specific auditory brainstem response, auditory steady-state response, new technologies in middle ear assessment, and advanced signal processing for hearing aids and cochlear implants.

Although the above technologies have advanced knowledge in the field of audiology, they raised new issues regarding the implementation of the new procedures and interpretation of test findings. In particular, assessing middle ear function in infants (aged 0 to 6 months) presents a new challenge to clinicians working in the field of pediatric diagnostic audiology. Variations in anatomy and physiology of the auditory system between infants and adults give rise to different middle ear dynamics, which in turn produce dissimilar test results, regardless of the technology used.

This book aims to provide a comprehensive overview of underpinning theoretical knowledge, clinical importance, latest research, and challenges in assessing the middle ear function of infants. As the first book of its kind, it will be a contemporary reference source for audiologists in training and clinicians, enabling them to make informed decisions about the middle ear status of infants. In addition to introducing the principles and protocols of middle ear assessments, case studies illustrating the application of the technologies to infants are provided.

The book begins with a chapter on the anatomy and physiology of the middle ear in infants, followed by an overview chapter on the applications of conventional tympanometry and stapedial acoustic reflex tests to infants and adults, including successes and failures. Chapter 3 provides a brief description of the principles of high-frequency (1 kHz) tympanometry, followed by an outline of the commonly used test protocols and interpretations of findings. The acoustic stapedial reflex test with a probe tone of 1 kHz, an important clinical test but rarely used with infants, is delineated in Chapter 4. Chapter 5 summarizes the current development of multifrequency tympanometry and its clinical applications. This chapter, drawing together elements from earlier chapters, provides further insight into middle ear dynamics in normal and pathological systems. Chapter 6 provides information on the engineering design and working principles of the sweep frequency impedance device. The successful application of this device to adults has led to the development of a new instrument for use with infants and neonates. Chapter 7 introduces the concept, principle, and clinical application of wideband acoustic transfer functions for evaluating middle ear function in both adults and infants. The last chapter provides a review of the different technologies, with emphasis on future directions in the instrumentation and their applications.

We are grateful to our colleagues who are dedicated to advancing our knowledge in this important area of assessing middle ear function in infants. We would also like to thank Professor Linda J. Hood for writing a Foreword for this book.

CONTRIBUTORS

M. Patrick Feeney, PhD
Director
VA RR&D National Center for
    Rehabilitative Auditory Research
Portland, OR
Affiliate Associate Professor
Department of Otolaryngology —
    Head and Neck Surgery
University of Washington
Seattle, WA
Chapter 7

Joseph Kei, PhD
Associate Professor
Head—Division of Audiology
Hearing Research Unit for Children
School of Health and Rehabilitation
    Sciences
University of Queensland
Queensland, Australia
Chapters 2, 3, 4, and 8

Rafidah Mazlan, PhD
Senior Lecturer
Department of Audiology and Speech
    Sciences
Faculty of Allied Health Sciences
Universiti Kebangsaan Malaysia
Kuala Lumpur, Malaysia
Chapters 2, 3, and 4

Michio Murakoshi, PhD
Assistant Professor
Department of Bioengineering and
    Robotics
Tohoku University
Sendai, Japan
Chapter 6

Chris A. Sanford, PhD
Assistant Professor
Department of Communication
    Sciences and Disorders
Idaho State University, ID
Chapter 7

Hiroshi Wada, PhD
Professor
Department of Bioengineering and
    Robotics
Tohoku University
Sendai, Japan
Chapter 6

Jie Wang, MD, PhD
Beijing Tongren Hospital
Capital Medical University
Beijing Institute of
    Otorhinolaryngology
Beijing, China
Chapter 5

Wayne Wilson, PhD
Senior Lecturer
Division of Audiology
Hearing Research Unit for Children
School of Health and Rehabilitation
    Sciences
The University of Queensland
    Queensland, Australia
Chapter 1

Fei Zhao, MD, PhD
Senior Lecturer
Director—Centre for Hearing and
    Balance Studies
University of Bristol
Bristol, United Kingdom
Chapters 5, 6, and 8

Anatomy and Physiology of the Outer and Middle Ear in Young Infants

WAYNE WILSON

INTRODUCTION

At the heart of any middle ear assessment are the outer and middle ear structures. Although much has been written about the embryology of these structures, surprisingly little has been written about their development after birth. With this in mind, this chapter reviews the anatomy and physiology of the outer and middle ear from birth to infancy in the human, with a particular emphasis on factors likely to affect middle ear assessment.

It is assumed that the reader has a basic understanding of the embryology of the outer and middle ear, and the anatomy and physiology of these structures in the adult human. All data presented in this chapter refer to human subjects (unless stated otherwise) born at full term. The terms *neonate* and *infant* are used to identify children aged 1 day to 4 weeks and 2 weeks to 36 months, respectively.

OUTER EAR AT BIRTH

The outer ear in the human is not completely mature at birth (Anson & Donaldson, 1981; Eby & Nadol, 1986; Qi, Funnell, & Daniel, 2008; Qi, Liu, Lutfy, Robert, Funnell, & Daniel, 2006; Saunders, Kaltenbach, & Relkin, 1983). Table 1–1 summarizes the major anatomical and physiological differences between the external auditory canals (EACs) of neonates versus adults based on published data.

TABLE 1–1. Summary of Neonate and Adult External Auditory Canal Data in the Human

External Auditory Canal (EAC)	Neonate	Adult
Shape	Straight[a]	S-shape[a]
Roof length (mm)	11–22.5[d]	25–30[b,c]
Floor length (mm)	17–22.5[d]	25–30[b,c]
Diameter (mm)	4.44[e]	10[b]
Bone	None[a]	Inner 2/3[b]
Soft tissue	Entire EAC[e]	Outer 1/3[a]
Does the EAC wall move with changes in EAC pressure?	Yes[f]	No[f]
Resonance frequency (kHz)	5.3–7.2[g]	2.7[g]

[a]Qi et al. (2006); [b]Saunders et al. (1983); [c]Stinson & Lawton (1989); [d]2-month-old neonate measurement (Mclellan & Webb, 1957); [e]Average ear canal diameter for 1-month-old neonate (Keefe et al., 1993); [f]Paradise et al. (1976) and Holte et al. (1990); [g]Kruger (1987).

Dimensions of the External Auditory Canal

The external auditory canal (EAC) of the neonate is straighter and approximately 50% shorter in length and diameter than that of the adult (although this percentage varies widely) (Keefe, Bulen, Arehart, & Burns, 1993; Mclellan & Webb, 1957; Qi et al., 2006; Saunders et al., 1983; Stinson & Lawton, 1989).

Compliance of the External Auditory Canal

In addition to the dimensional differences between the EAC of the neonate and the adult is the finding that almost the entire EAC of the neonate is surrounded by soft tissue, compared to only the outer third of the EAC in the adult (the inner two-thirds being surrounded by the temporal bone) (Mclellan & Webb, 1957).

The soft tissue that surrounds the EAC in both neonates and adults is a thin layer of cartilage, or more specifically, elastic cartilage (as versus articular or fibrocartilage) (Fung, 1993; Mclellan & Webb, 1957). Elastic cartilage contains many elastic fibers made up of type II collagen (as does, to a lesser extent, articular cartilage), making it highly compliant (Anson & Donaldson, 1981) and the most flexible of the cartilage types in humans (Fung, 1993).

The compliance of neonate elastic cartilage has not been measured, although Qi et al. (2006) used three Young's moduli (i.e., 30, 60, and 90 kPa) in their nonlinear finite-element model of the neonate ear canal. The 30-kPa value was close to the lowest stiffness of soft tissue such as fat (4.8 kPa) and gland (17.5 kPa) (Wellman et al., 1999 cited in Qi et al., 2006). The 90-kPa value was close to the lowest stiffness of cartilage in adults (between 100 kPa and 1 MPa) (Liu, Kerdok, & Howe, 2004, cited in Qi et al., 2006; Zhang, Zheng, & Mak, 1997). (Note: Young's modulus is a measure of stiffness, defined as the ratio of uniaxial stress over uniaxial strain when the range of stress satisfies Hooke's law. As stress is measured in pascals and strain is dimensionless, Young's modulus is measured in pascals. The higher the value of Young's modulus, the higher the stiffness of the material being measured [for example, estimates of Young's modulus for rubber can be in the range of 10 to 100 MPa, and for diamond can be greater than 1000 GPa.])

The low stiffness of the walls of the neonate EAC suggests that these walls could move if the air pressure in the EAC was changed. Such movement was observed by Paradise, Smith, and Bluestone (1976), who reported significantly greater EAC wall distensibility in neonates versus subjects aged one year or over. Paradise et al.'s (1976) study had been limited, however, by their use of a subjective rating based on a visual inspection of canal wall distensibility during pneumatic otoscopy. Later, Cavanaugh (1989) noted that the pressure changes induced by pneumatic otoscopy in the EAC of infants, children, and adolescents was highly variable, ranging from 338 to 1134 mm H_2O. Holte, Cavanaugh, and Margolis (1990) subsequently noted that these pressures were significantly higher than those typically induced during tympanometry (± 250 to 300 daPa). These authors went on to video record the EAC walls of 36 ears in neonates aged 1 to 7 days as the pressure in their EACs was changed by mechanically controlled pneumatic otos-

copy. By reviewing the video tapes of the EACs during these pressure changes (with the aid of a transparent ruler and a video enhancer), they reported average changes in the diameter of the EAC (from rest) of 18.3% and −28.2 % in response to positive and negative air pulses of ± 250 to 300 daPa, respectively. These results show that the walls of the EAC in neonates can move if the air pressure in the EAC is changed, even within the range typically induced by tympanometry.

Resonance Frequency of the External Auditory Canal

The resonance frequency of the EAC is inversely proportional to its length. Hence, the resonance frequency of the EAC for infants will be higher than that for adults (*Note:* According to ANSI [2009] ASA S2.1-2009/ISO 2041: *American National Standard Mechanical Vibration, Shock and Condition Monitoring-Vocabulary*, the term "resonance frequency" should be used rather than "resonant frequency."). Kruger (1987) determined diffuse field to ear canal sound pressure transformation in children from birth to 3 years of age. She noted that the EAC fundamental resonance frequency for children ranged from approximately 5.3 to 7.2 kHz, which was about 2 to 3 times higher than that of adults (approximately 2.7 kHz).

Appearance of the External Auditory Canal on Otoscopy

One of the more detailed descriptions of the appearance of the neonate EAC during otoscopy is offered by Mclellan and

Webb (1957). On inspecting the natural appearance of the EACs in 204 ears of 102 neonates less than 24 hours old, these authors found varying amounts of white or grayish-white, semisolid, creamy material in every ear. They assumed that this material was the same as the vernix caseosa on the skin of the neonates. The amount of vernix varied, depending on the individual. In some cases, it filled the EAC almost completely. These authors also inspected the natural appearance of the EACs in 20 of their subjects after these EACs had been cleaned. In these clean EACs, they noted no visible cerumen; hairs (with one subject having enough hairs to block vision of the tympanic membrane); shorter superior walls than inferior walls; poorly defined junctions between the EACs and the pars flaccida; a peaking of the inferior walls to form a transverse ridge at their midpoints, which created an outer hairy part and an inner, smooth, glabrous part in each EAC; and wider superior and inferior walls than anterior and posterior walls, the latter two walls appearing curved in sagittal cross-section.

DEVELOPMENT OF THE OUTER EAR FROM BIRTH TO INFANCY

Dimensions of the External Auditory Canal

The diameter and length of the EAC increase significantly from birth through 12 months of age, with authors such as Keefe et al. (1993) reporting that the average EAC diameter increased from 4.4 mm to 7.0 mm, and the average EAC length increased from 14.0 mm to 20.0 mm in 88 subjects as they aged from 1 to 12 months. These and other authors note that further increases will continue until approximately 9 years of age where adultlike diameters of approximately 10 mm, lengths of approximately 25 mm, and increased degrees of curvature of the EAC are achieved (Abdala & Keefe, 2006; Keefe et al., 1993; Wright, 1997).

Compliance of the External Auditory Canal

In addition to the dimensional differences, the mechanical properties of the cartilage surrounding the EAC change, as does the proportion of the EAC surrounded by cartilage. Although the compliance of the elastic cartilage of a neonate has not been measured, its mechanical properties are thought to be age dependent, with Williamson, Chen, and Sah (2001) finding the Young's modulus of bovine articular cartilage increases by an average of 275% from neonate to adult. With regard to the proportion of the EAC surrounded by cartilage, this decreases rapidly from birth through to 12 months of age (Anson, Bast, & Richany, 1955; Anson & Donaldson, 1981). By this stage, the EAC is approaching its adultlike state in that its outer third is surrounded by cartilage whereas its inner two-thirds is surrounded by the temporal bone.

The increased proportion of the bony part of the EAC leads to an increased stiffness in the walls of this canal. This affects the movement of these walls if the air pressure in the EAC is changed. After reporting changes in the diameter of the EAC (from rest) of 18.3% and −28.2% in response to positive and negative air pulses of ±250 to 300 daPa, respectively, in their subjects aged 1 to 7 days, Holte et al. (1990) reported changes of only 7.9 % and −15.0% (respectively) in their subjects at 11 to 22 days, 2.9% and −6.4% (respectively) in their subjects aged 26 to 47 days, 0% and −1.5% (respectively) in their subjects aged 51 to 66 days, and 0% and 0% (respectively) in their subjects aged 103 to 133 days. These authors concluded that changes in air pressure during tympanometry do not cause the EAC walls to move in children aged 56 days and above.

Resonance Frequency of the External Auditory Canal

As the length of the EAC increases from birth to infancy, the resonance frequency decreases in view of the inverse relationship between the two measures. Kruger (1987) and Bentler (1989) showed that the initially high resonance frequency (5.3 to 7.2 kHz) of the EAC at birth reported by Kruger (1987) decreases with age to reach adultlike values (approximately 2.7 kHz) by the second year of life.

MIDDLE EAR AT BIRTH

The middle ear in the human is not completely mature at birth (Eby & Nadol, 1986; Qi et al., 2006; Saunders et al.,

1983). Table 1–2 summarizes the major anatomical and physiological differences between the middle ears of neonates versus adults based on published data.

Tympanic Cavity

Early reports suggested that the tympanic cavity reaches adult size at birth (Anson, Bast, & Cauldwell, 1948; Anson, Cauldwell, & Bast, 1948) with only a smaller distance noted between the stapes footplate and the tympanic membrane (TM) (Eby & Nadol, 1986). More recent data, however, suggest that, although the bony configuration of the tympanic cavity within the petrous bone is established by the time of birth (Anson et al., 1955), the volume of the tympanic cavity is actually smaller in neonates than in adults. Ikui, Sando, Haginomori, and Sudo (2000) reported that the average volume of the tympanic cavity in infants less than 1 year was 452 mm^3 (with the one subject aged less than 1 week showing a volume of approximately 400 mm^3) compared to 640 mm^3 in adults.

Temporal bone studies of the contents of the tympanic cavity at birth have regularly indicated the presence of mesenchyme, middle ear effusion and other material (Anson et al., 1955). In a study of the tympanic space in 111 temporal bones of infants aged 0 to 2 years, Paparella, Shea, Meyerhoff, and Goycoolea (1980) found many cases of marked mesenchymal tissue retention, whereas de Sa (1973) found amniotic fluid or mucoid effusion in the tympanic space of 60% of 130 temporal bones

TABLE 1–2. Summary of Neonate and Adult Middle Ear Data in the Human

Structure	Aspect	Neonate	Adult
Tympanic membrane	Diameter along manubrium (mm)	8–10[a]	8–10[a]
	Diameter perpendicular to manubrium (mm)	7–9[a]	7–9[a]
	Surface area (mm^2)	55–85[a]	55–85[a]
	Thickness of pars tensa (mm)	0.1–1.5[b]	0.04–0.12[c]
	Vascular and cellular content	More[b]	Less[b]
	Collagen and elastin fibres	Less[b]	More[b]
	Plane, relative to EAC axis (horizontal)	Nearly horizontal[d,e]	Approx. 45°[d,e]
	Tympanic ring	Unfused[f]	Fused[f]
Tympanic cavity	Volume (mm^3)	452[d]	640[d]
	Presence of mesenchyme, effusion and other material	Yes[b]	No[b]
Ossicles	Formation and ossification	Possibly incomplete	Complete
Middle ear muscles	Development	Complete[a,e,f]	Complete[a,e,f]
Eustachian tube	Efficiency	Inefficient	Efficient
Middle ear as a whole	Resonance frequency (Hz)	450 and 710[g]	800–1200[h]
	Input admittance	Smaller in magnitude, dominated by mass and/or resistance[g,h]	Larger in magnitude, dominated by stiffness[g,h]

[a]Saunders et al. (1983); [b]Ruah et al. (1991); [c]Kuypers et al. (2006); [d]Infants less than 1 year old (Mclellan & Webb, 1957); [e]Qi et al. (2006); [f]Anson et al. (1955); [g]Holte et al. (1991); [h]Homma et al. (2009).

of neonates. In reviewing more recent reports, Hsu, Margolis, and Schachern (2000) noted reports of foreign material, including blood, exudate, desquamated epithelium, hair, and inflammatory cells in neonate and infant temporal bones; the universal presence of subepithelial mesenchyme in neonate temporal bones (Piza, Northrop, & Eavey, 1996); cases where mesenchyme occupied much of the middle ear space and was in contact with the ossicles in neonates (Eavey, 1993); blood and purulent otitis media (OM) in the tympanic cavity of neonates

(Eavey, 1993); and reports that cellular content is more likely to be present in the tympanic cavity when the neonate is born through meconium-contaminated amniotic fluid (Piza, Gonzalez, Northrop, & Eavey, 1989). Many of the temporal bone studies must be considered with caution, however, as they often involve cases of neonate death and systemic infection.

Tympanic Membrane

The tympanic membrane is adult size at birth (Qi et al., 2006). At this stage it already contains all three major layers: the outer layer or epidermis, with an ultrastructure similar to the epidermis of skin; the middle layer or lamina propria, which contains a loose ground matrix and two layers of densely packed collagen arranged in radial and circular patterns, respectively; and the thin inner layer or lamina mucosa, which contains a large number of columnar cells (Lim, 1970). The ultrastructure of the TM in neonates is not completely adultlike, however, with electron microscopy by Ruah Schachern, Zelterman, Paparella, and Yoon (1991) showing the TMs in neonates to be more vascular, more cellular, and having less collagen and elastins than in adults.

The thickness of the TM in the neonate has not been widely studied. Using histological images and light and electron microscopy, Ruah et al. (1991) estimated TM thicknesses in neonates to range from 0.4 to 0.7 mm in the posterior-superior quadrant; 0.1 to 0.25 mm in the posterior-inferior, anterior-supe-

rior and anterior-inferior quadrants; and from 0.7 to 1.5 mm near the umbo. Qi et al. (2008) supplemented these findings with thickness measurements on histological images from two one-month-old ears to derive a nonuniform thickness of 0.1 mm for the posterior-inferior, anterior-superior, and anterior-inferior quadrants; 0.5 mm for the posterior-superior quadrant; and 0.75 mm near the umbo (excluding the manubrium). These thickness values in neonates generally were larger than the 0.04 to 0.12-mm thickness values reported by Kuypers, Decraemer, and Dirckx (2006) for the central region of the pars tensa in three adults; and the 0.03 to 0.23 mm for the pars flacida and 0.03 to 0.09 mm for the pars tensa reported by Lim (1970) and Schmidt and Hellstrom (1991).

The compliance of the TM in the neonate depends mainly on its middle layer, the lamina propria. This layer is characterized by the presence of type II collagen (Qi et al., 2008; Ruah et al., 1991), with the mechanical properties of collagen being mostly decided by its density, length, cross-linking, and the diameters and orientations of its fibers. To date, the Young's modulus of the neonate TM has not been thoroughly investigated, and no direct measurements of the mechanical properties of the TM in neonates are available. Qi et al. (2008) noted that the age-related Young's modulus of another collagen containing membrane and skin, was found by Rollhauser (1950) (cited in Qi et al., 2008), to be 7 to 8 times smaller in 3-month-old infants than in adults. Similar results were reported by Yamada (1970). With this in mind, Qi et al.

(2008) used three Young's moduli for the neonate TM in their study: 0.6, 1.2 and 2.4 MPa. They reported these values as being consistent with the adult to infant ratios of 6 to 8 found by Rollhauser (1950) (cited in Qi et al. [2008] and Yamada [1970]) with 0.6 MPa being several times smaller than Decraemer, Maes, and Vanhuyse's (1980) typical small-strain modulus value, and 2.4 MPa being approximately 8 to 10 times smaller than both Decraemer, Maes, and Vanhuyse's (1980) typical large-strain modulus value and the measurement of Békésy (1960).

As with the tympanic membrane, the tympanic ring is also immature at birth. At this stage, its superior aspect (at the tympanic incisure or notch of Rivinus) is still partially open, showing only localized fusion to the squamous part of the temporal bone. Its inner surface is also typically grooved by the tympanic sulcus for the attachment of the tympanic membrane, and the tympanic tubercles may be evident as two bulges of the ring (Anson et al., 1955; Humphrey & Scheuer, 2006).

Middle Ear Ossicles

The status of the middle ear ossicles at birth is disputed. Some authors claim that the ossicles are completely formed and ossified prior to birth (Anson et al., 1955; Bast, 1942; Saunders et al., 1983). Other authors have reported that, compared to adults, the ossicles in neonates are smaller in weight and size (Olszewski, 1990); have longer, narrower anterior mallear processes (Anson & Donaldson, 1981; Qi et al., 2008; Unur, Ülger, & Ekinci, 2002); have more bone marrow in the malleus and incus (Yokoyama, Iino, Kakizaki, & Murakami, 1999); have looser osscular joints (Anson & Donaldson, 1981); and have tighter coupling between the stapes and annular ligament (Keefe et al., 1993). The orientation of the middle ear ossicles is also likely to be influenced by the smaller volume of the middle ear cavity at birth (Abdala & Keefe, 2006).

Appearance of the Tympanic Membrane and Ossicles During Otoscopy

One of the more detailed descriptions of the appearance of the neonate TM and ossicles during otoscopy is offered by Mclellan and Webb (1957). These authors inspected the appearance of the TM and tympanic cavity after cleaning the external auditory canals in 102 ears of 51 neonates less than 24 hours old. They found that the pars tensa was gray in 16.7% of ears, pink in 70.6% of ears, and red in 12.7% of ears; the pars flacida was gray in 1.0% of ears, pink in 31.4% of ears and red in 67.6% or ears; the cone of light was seen on the TM in 26.5% of ears; the short process of the malleus was the dominant aspect of the ossicles and was seen through the TM in 100% of ears; and the TMs were well seen in 100% of ears. Overall, Mclellan and Webb (1957) described the TMs of their subjects as being dull, red, thickened, and retracted with poorly defined landmarks. They noted that by adult standards, all of the TMs they observed would have been classified as abnormal.

Middle Ear Muscles

The stapedius and tensor tympani muscles of the middle ear are reported to be fully developed prior to birth (Anson et al., 1955; Qi et al., 2006; Saunders et al., 1983). This leaves these muscles able to contribute to their respective reflexes, assuming the remainder of the acoustic reflex pathway is intact and functioning normally. Clear evidence from Mazlan, Kei, and Hickson (2009) shows that acoustic stapedial reflex was present in 91.3% of 219 neonates in the well-baby nursery. The remaining 8.7% of neonates had auditory disorders as confirmed by otoacoustic emission and high-frequency tympanometry results.

Eustachian Tube

The eustachian tube in the neonate differs significantly from the eustachian tube in the adult. It is shorter, has a less well-defined isthmus, is almost horizontal (lying on an angle of approximately 10°), has its nasopharyngeal opening located closer to the level of the soft palate (leaving it more exposed as it lies lower in the shallower nasopharyngeal vault), and is surrounded by considerably more glandular tissue. Its tubal cartilage is also farther away from the levator palate muscle (rendering this muscle ineffective) and can only be acted upon by the tensor palate muscle. Although the eustachian tube in the neonate may open sharply, it often closes more gradually. These anatomical and physiological differences result in a general tubal inefficiency in the neonate (Holborow, 1970, 1975; Holmquist, 1977; Proctor, 1967).

Resonance and Admittance of the Middle Ear

Using multifrequency tympanometry, Holte, Margolis, and Cavanaugh (1991) found two resonant peaks in the middle ears of neonates: one at about 450 Hz and one at about 710 Hz. Both of these middle ear resonant frequencies are significantly lower than that of the adult, which occurs at around 0.8 to 1.2 kHz (Homma, Du, Shimizu, & Puria, 2009).

The input admittance of the neonate middle ear is smaller in magnitude and dominated by mass and/or resistance compared to the input admittance of the adult middle ear, which is larger in magnitude and dominated by stiffness (Holte et al., 1991; Homma et al., 2009; Purdy & Williams, 2000). One possible reason for the dominant mass and/or resistance components in the neonate is the presence of material other than air in the tympanic cavity (discussed above), which could add mass to the ossicular chain (Holte et al., 1991).

DEVELOPMENT OF THE MIDDLE EAR FROM BIRTH TO INFANCY

Tympanic Cavity

Early reports claimed little growth of the tympanic cavity in the first 6 months of life, with changes in the angle of the planes of the TM and the skull base merely increasing the distance from the stapes footplate to the TM (Eby & Nadol, 1986). Later reports claimed more extensive growth, with Ikui et al. (2000) finding the average volume of the tympanic cavity increased by approximately 1.5 times from birth to adulthood (from 451.7 ± 6.82 mm^3 to 640.1 ± 69.1 mm^3). These authors observed the greatest enlargement in the hypotympanum (2.5 to 3.2 times) followed by the epitympanum (1.9 to 2.1 times) and the mesotympanum (1.1 to 1.2 times). Much of this increase in volume was driven by a 1.2 to 1.4 times increase in the height of the tympanic cavity, with more vertical growth observed in the epitympanum and hypotympanum (as the mastoid and mandible developed) than in the mesotympanum. This increase in the volume of the tympanic cavity also correlated with this cavity's degree of pneumatization.

The postnatal increase in tympanic cavity volume is accompanied by an increase in the pneumatisation and growth of temporal bone as a whole, particularly the mastoid process (Anson et al., 1955). Anson et al. (1955) reported the pneumatization of the temporal bone as being an extension of the pneumatisation of the tympanic cavity and antrum that began prior to birth. Eby and Nadol (1986) reported growths in the mastoid portion of the temporal bone from 1 year to adulthood of 2.0 to 2.6 cm in length, 1.7 cm in width, and 0.8 to 0.9 cm in depth. As the mastoid air cells are continuous with the middle ear cavity, both the pneumatization and the growth of these spaces could contribute to the increasing volume of the complex middle ear space (Holte et al., 1991).

The mesenchyme, middle ear effusion and other material present reported in the neonate's tympanic cavity (Anson et al., 1955; de Sa, 1973; Hsu et al., 2000; Paparella et al., 1980) may persist well into the child's development. Anson et al. (1955) claimed that mesenchyme may persist in the tympanic space up to 5 months after birth, whereas Crowe and Polvogt (1930) and Paparella et al. (1980) reported unresolved mesenchyme in the temporal bones of adults. Paparella et al. (1980) and Kasemsuwan, Schachern, Paparella, and Le (1996) cited the presence of unresolved mesenchyme as a potential contributor in the pathogenesis of otitis media. Anson et al. (1955) also noted that as the mesenchyme is absorbed by the tympanic cavity, the air space in this cavity expands. This expanding air space can be increased when coupled with possible growth of the tympanic cavity, especially in the first few postnatal months (Bast, 1930).

Tympanic Membrane

The thickness of the TM decreases significantly from birth to adulthood (Ruah et al., 1991), with the TM becoming less vascular and less cellular, and developing more collagen fibers and elastins (Ruah et al., 1991). Although the exact changes in the collagen fibres of the TM have not been directly studied, other collagen fibres in the body have been shown to increase their length (Qi et al., 2008), density and number of crosslinks, and become more aligned, with age (Hall, 1976; Stoltz, 2006). Similarly, although age-related changes to Young's modulus in the TM have not been reported, Young's modulus in human skin has been shown to increase by approximately 7 to 8 times from 3 months of age to adulthood (Yamada, 1970). The shape of the tympanic membrane may also assume a more conical shape as the child ages. This change accounts for the change in the shape of the light reflex from short and wide to pie-shaped during childhood (Anson et al., 1955).

A more dramatic change in the tympanic membrane occurs as a result of changes in the temporal bone and the tympanic ring. Soon after birth, during the fusion of several different parts of the temporal bone, the inferior section of the tympanic ring fuses to the lower border of the tympanic cavity (Humphrey & Scheuer, 2006). As the first year of life progresses, two bony prominences (the anterior and posterior tympanic tubercles) grow across the ring and fuse together to form a second aperture separate to the EAC, the foramen of Huschke. This foramen closes as the tubercles grow in from its edges (although it can remain patent in some subjects, with incidences ranging from 0 to 67%) (Anson et al., 1955; Humphrey & Scheuer, 2006). At the same time, the tympanic plate of the temporal bone extends laterally to convert the original tympanic ring into the bony EAC (Dahm, Shepherd, & Clark, 1993). This lateral growth causes a considerable change in the orientation of the plane of the tympanic membrane from its nearly horizontal position at birth to the 30 to 45° (the adult position) by four to five years of age (Anson et al., 1955; Eby & Nadol, 1986; Ikui, Sando, Sudo, & Fujita, 1997; Qi et al., 2006).

Middle Ear Ossicles

Just as the status of the ossicles at birth is disputed, so too is their development after birth. In support of continuing ossicular development are reports of increases in ossicular weight and size (Olszewski, 1990); changes in the long, narrow anterior mallear process (Anson & Donaldson, 1981; Qi et al., 2008; Unur et al., 2002); the replacement of bone marrow with bone in the malleus and incus, with full ossification achieved by approximately 25 months of age; tightening of the ossicular joints (Anson & Donaldson, 1981); looser coupling between the stapes and annular ligament (Keefe et al., 1993); and changes in tympanic membrane orientation leading to changes in ossicular orientation, particularly the manubrium (Anson, Cauldwell, & Bast, 1948). Finally, the bone of the ossicles is thought to be remodelled and may become pneumatized after birth (Anson et al., 1955; Richany, Bast, & Anson, 1954).

Eustachian Tube

The eustachian tube develops slowly, taking approximately seven years to reach adultlike levels of structure and function. By that stage, it will have increased in length from 30 mm to 40 mm, formed a well-defined isthmus, increased its angle to the horizontal plain to approximately 45°, had its nasopharyngeal opening move away from the level of the soft palate (reducing this opening's exposure to the nasopharyngeal vault), and become less surrounded by glandular tissue. Its tubal cartilage will also be closer to the levator palate muscle (allowing both this muscle and the tensor palate muscle to act on this cartilage) and it will be better able to open and close sharply. These anatomical and physiological changes result in a general tubal efficiency from the age of approximately seven years and above (Holborow, 1970, 1975; Holmquist, 1977; Proctor, 1967).

Resonance and Admittance of the Middle Ear

The middle ear resonance frequencies of neonates (one at about 450 Hz and one at about 710 Hz) increase with age to 0.8 to 1.2 kHz by 4 to 7 months of age (Holte et al., 1991; Homma et al., 2009; Purdy & Williams, 2000).

The smaller magnitude input admittance that is mass and/or resistance dominated in the middle ears of neonates, becomes a larger magnitude input admittance that is stiffness dominated in the middle ears of subjects from approximately 4 to 7 months of age and beyond (Holte et al., 1991; Homma et al., 2009; Keefe et al., 1993; Keefe, Fitzpatrick, Liu, Sanford, & Gorga, 2010; Purdy & Williams, 2000). A possible reason for the increase in admittance magnitude is the growth of the tympanic cavity (discussed above), as input admittance increases with the size of a volume of air (Holte et al., 1991).

CONCLUSION

The above literature review indicates that outer and middle ears in the neonate are not completely mature at birth, with some components taking weeks and others taking years to mature. In general, there is an increase in dimensions and a change in the relative positioning of the components of the auditory system. In turn, these changes may alter the acoustical properties and dynamics of the outer and middle ears, resulting in dissimilar assessment findings when compared to those obtained from adults. The maturational elements most likely to affect the assessment of middle ear function in neonates and infants include:

- The decrease in resonance frequency of the EAC, due primarily to its increase in length.

- The increase in stiffness of the EAC, due to the formation of its bony canal wall.

- The increase in size of the tympanic cavity.

- The decrease in the overall mass and resistance of the middle ear, due (at least in part) to loss of mesenchyme and changes in bone density of the ossicles.

- The increase in overall stiffness of the middle ear, due (at least in part) to changes in the orientation and fiber content of the tympanic membrane, fusion of the tympanic ring, and tightening of the ossicular joints.

- The increase in the resonance frequency of the middle ear, due to the decrease in its mass and increase in its stiffness.

With these maturation elements in mind, it is clear that the valid and reliable measurement of middle ear function in neonates and infants may require tools and protocols beyond those used to assess middle ear function in adults.

REFERENCES

Abdala, C., & Keefe, D. H. (2006). Effects of middle-ear immaturity on distortion product otoacoustic emission suppression tuning in infant ears. *Journal of the Acoustical Society of America, 120*(6), 3832–3842.

American National Standards Institute (ANSI). (2009). *American National Standard Mechanical Vibration, Shock and Condition Monitoring—Vocabulary.* ASA S2.1-2009/ISO 2041:2009. New York, NY: Author.

(Anson, B. J., Bast, H., & Richany, S. F. (1955). The fetal and early postnatal development of the tympanic ring and related structures in man. *Annals of Otology, Rhinology, and Larynogology, 64,* 802–823.

Anson, B. J., Bast, T. H., & Cauldwell, E. W. (1948). The development of the auditory ossicles, the otic capsule and the extracapsular tissues. *Annals of Otology, Rhinology, and Laryngology, 57*(3), 603–632.

Anson, B. J., Cauldwell, E. W., & Bast, T. H. (1948). The fissula ante fenestram of the human otic capsule II. Aberrant form and contents. *Annals of Otology, Rhinology, and Laryngology, 57*(1), 103–128.

Anson, B. J., & Donaldson, J. A. (1981). *Surgical anatomy of the temporal bone and ear.* Philadelphia, PA: Saunders.

Bast, T. H. (1930). Ossification of the otic capsule in human fetuses. *Contributions to Embryology, 21,* 53–82.

Bast, T. H. (1942). Development of the otic capsule. VI. Histological changes and variations in the growing bony capsule of the vestibule and cochlea. *Annals of Otology, Rhinology, and Laryngology, 51,* 343–357.

Békésy, G. V. (1960). *Experiments in hearing.* New York, NY: AIP Press.

Bentler, R. A. (1989). External ear resonance characteristics in children. *Journal of Speech and Hearing Disorders, 54*(2), 264–268.

Cavanaugh, R. M., Jr. (1989). Pediatricians and the pneumatic otoscope: Are we playing it by ear? *Pediatrics, 84*(2), 362–364.

Crowe, S. J., & Polvogt, L. M. (1930). Embryonic tissue in the middle ear and mastoid —Report of two cases. *Journal of Otolaryngology, 12*(2), 151–161.

Dahm, M. C., Shepherd, R. K., & Clark, G. M. (1993). The postnatal-growth of the temporal bone and its implications for cochlear implantation in children. *Acta Oto-Laryngologica Supplementum, 505,* 1–39.

de Sa, D. J. (1973). Infection and amniotic aspiration of middle ear in stillbirths and neonatal deaths. *Archives of Disease in Children, 48*(11), 872–880.

Decraemer, W. F., Maes, M. A., & Vanhuyse, V. J. (1980). An elastic stress-strain relation for soft biological tissues based on a structural model. *Journal of Biomechanics, 13*(6), 463–468.

Eavey, R. D. (1993). Abnormalities of the neonatal ear: otoscopic observations, histologic observations, and a model for contamination of the middle ear by cellular contents of amniotic fluid. *Laryngoscope, 103*(1 Pt. 2, Suppl. 58), 1–31.

Eby, T. L., & Nadol, J. B., Jr. (1986). Postnatal growth of the human temporal bone: Implications for cochlear implants in children. *Annals of Otology, Rhinology, and Laryngology, 95*(4 Pt. 1), 356–364.

Fung, Y. C. (1993). *Biomechanics: Mechanical properties of living tissues* (2nd ed.), Berlin, Germany: Springer-Verlag.

Hall, D. A. (1976). *The aging of connective tissue.* London, UK: Academic.

Holborow, C. (1970). Eustachian tubal function—Changes in anatomy and function with age and relationship of these changes to aural pathology. *Archives of Otolaryngology, 92*(6), 624–626.

Holborow, C. (1975). Eustachian tubal function—Changes throughout childhood and neuromuscular control. *Journal of Laryngology and Otology, 89*(1), 47–55.

Holmquist, J. (1977). Eustachian tube anatomy and physiology. *Journal of the American Audiology Society, 2*(4), 115–120.

Holte, L., Cavanaugh, R. M., & Margolis, R. H. (1990). Ear canal wall mobility and tympanometric shape in young infants. *Journal of Pediatrics, 117*(1), 77–80.

Holte, L., Margolis, R. H., & Cavanaugh, R. M. (1991). Developmental changes in multifrequency tympanograms. *Audiology, 30*(1), 1–24.

Homma, K., Du, Y., Shimizu, Y., & Puria, S. (2009). Ossicular resonance modes of the human middle ear for bone and air conduction. *Journal of the Acoustical Society of America, 125*(2), 968–979.

Hsu, G. S., Margolis, R. H., & Schachern, P. A. (2000). Development of the middle ear in neonatal chinchillas. I. Birth to 13 days. *Acta Oto-Laryngologica, 120*(8), 922–932.

Humphrey, L. T., & Scheuer, L. (2006). Age of closure of the foramen of Huschke: An osteological study. *International Journal of Osteoarchaeology, 16*(1), 47–60.

Ikui, A., Sando, I., Haginomori, S., & Sudo, M. (2000). Postnatal development of the tympanic cavity: A computer-aided reconstruction and measurement study. *Acta Oto-Laryngologica, 120*(3), 375–379.

Ikui, A., Sando, I., Sudo, M., & Fujita, S. (1997). Postnatal change in angle between the tympanic annulus and surrounding structures: Computer-aided three-dimensional reconstruction study. *Annals of Otology, Rhinology, and Laryngology, 106*(1), 33–36.

Kasemsuwan, L., Schachern, P., Paparella, M. M., & Le, C. T. (1996). Residual mesenchyme in temporal bones of children. *Laryngoscope, 106*(8), 1040–1043.

Keefe, D. H., Bulen, J. C., Arehart, K. H., & Burns, E. M. (1993). Ear-canal impedance and reflection coefficient in human infants and adults. *Journal of the Acoustical Society of America, 94*(5), 2617–2638.

Keefe, D. H., Fitzpatrick, D., Liu, Y. W., Sanford, C. A., & Gorga, M. P. (2010). Wideband acoustic-reflex test in a test battery to predict middle-ear dysfunction. *Hearing Research, 263*(1–2), 52–65.

Kruger, B. (1987). An update on the external ear resonance in infants and young children. *Ear and Hearing, 8*(6), 333–336.

Kuypers, L. C., Decraemer, W. F., & Dirckx, J. J. (2006). Thickness distribution of fresh and preserved human eardrums measured with confocal microscopy. *Otology and Neurotology, 27*(2), 256–264.

Lim, D. J. (1970). Human tympanic membrane. An ultrastructural observation. *Acta Oto-Laryngologica, 70*(3), 176–186.

Liu, Y., Kerdok, A. E., & Howe, R. D. (2004). A nonlinear finite element model of soft tissue indentation. *Proceedings of medical simulation: International symposium* (pp. 67–76). Cambridge, MA: Springer-Verlag.

Mazlan, R., Kei, J., & Hickson, L. (2009). Test-retest reliability of acoustic reflex testing in healthy newborns. *Ear and Hearing, 30*, 295–301.

Mclellan, M. S., & Webb, C. H. (1957). Ear studies in the newborn infant—Natural appearance and incidence of obscuring by vernix, cleansing of vernix, and description of drum and canal after cleansing. *Journal of Pediatrics, 51*(6), 672–677.

Olszewski, J. (1990). Zur Morphometrie der Gehöknöchelchen beim Menschen im Rahmen der Entwicklung [The morphometry of the ear ossicles in humans during development]. *Anatomischer Anzeiger, 171*(3), 187–191.

Paparella, M. M., Shea, D., Meyerhoff, W. L., & Goycoolea, M. V. (1980). Silent otitis media. *Laryngoscope, 90*(7 Pt. 1), 1089–1098.

Paradise, J. L., Smith, C. G., & Bluestone, C. D. (1976). Tympanometric detection of middle ear effusion in infants and young children. *Pediatrics, 58*(2), 198–210.

Piza, J., Gonzalez, M., Northrop, C. C., & Eavey, R. D. (1989). Meconium contamination of the neonatal middle ear. *Journal of Pediatrics, 115*(6), 910–914.

Piza, J. E., Northrop, C. C., & Eavey, R. D. (1996). Neonatal mesenchyme temporal bone study: Typical receding pattern versus increase in Potter's sequence. *Laryngoscope, 106*(7), 856–864.

Proctor, B. (1967). Embryology and anatomy of eustachian tube. *Archives of Otolaryngology, 86*(5), 503–507.

Purdy, S. C., & Williams, M. J. (2000). High frequency tympanometry: A valid and reliable immittance test protocol for young infants? *New Zealand Audiological Society Bulletin, 10*, 9–24.

Qi, L., Funnell, W. R. J., & Daniel, S. J. (2008). A nonlinear finite-element model of the newborn middle ear. *Journal of the Acoustical Society of America, 124*(1), 337–347.

Qi, L., Liu, H. J., Lutfy, J., Robert, W., Funnell, J., & Daniel, S. J. (2006). A nonlinear finite-element model of the newborn ear canal. *Journal of the Acoustical Society of America, 120*(6), 3789–3798.

Richany, S. F., Bast, T. H., & Anson, B. J. (1954). The development and adult structure of the malleus, incus and stapes. *Annals of Otology, Rhinology, and Laryngology, 63*(2), 394–434.

Ruah, C. B., Schachern, P. A., Zelterman, D., Paparella, M. M., & Yoon, T. H. (1991). Age-related morphologic changes in the human tympanic membrane. A light and electron microscopic study. *Archives of Otolaryngology-Head and Neck Surgery, 117*(6), 627–634.

Saunders, J. C., Kaltenbach, J. A., & Relkin, E. M. (1983). The structural and functional development of the outer and middle ear. In R. Romand & R. Marty (Eds.), *Development of auditory and vestibular systems*. New York, NY: Academic.

Schmidt, S. H., & Hellstrom, S. (1991). Tympanic-membrane structure—new views: A comparative study. *ORL Journal for Oto-Rhino-Laryngology, 53*(1), 32–36.

Stinson, M. R., & Lawton, B. W. (1989). Specification of the geometry of the human ear canal for the prediction of sound-pressure level distribution. *Journal of the Acoustical Society of America, 85*(6), 2492–2503.

Stoltz, J. F. (2006). *Mechanobiology: Cartilage and chondrocytes* (Vol. 4). Washington, DC: IOS Press.

Unur, E., Ülger, H., & Ekinci, N. (2002). Morphometrical and morphological variations of middle ear ossicles in the newborn. *Erciyes Medical Journal, 24*, 57–63.

Williamson, A. K., Chen, A. C., & Sah, R. L. (2001). Compressive properties and function—Composition relationships of developing bovine articular cartilage. *Journal of Orthopaedic Research, 19*(6), 1113–1121.

Wright, C. G. (1997). Development of the human external ear. *Journal of the American Academy of Audiology, 8*(6), 379–382.

Yamada, H. (1970). *Strength of biological materials*. Baltimore, MD: Williams and Wilkins.

Yokoyama, T., Iino, Y., Kakizaki, K., & Murakami, Y. (1999). Human temporal bone study on the postnatal ossification process of auditory ossicles. *Laryngoscope, 109*(6), 927–930.

Zhang M., Zheng, Y. P., & Mak, A. F. (1997). Estimating the effective Young's modules of soft tissues from identation test—Nonlinear finite element analysis of effects of friction and large deformation. *Medical Engineering and Physics, 19*(6), 512–517.

CHAPTER 2

Measuring Middle Ear Function in Young Infants: An Overview

RAFIDAH MAZLAN AND JOSEPH KEI

INTRODUCTION

This chapter provides a brief review of the literature regarding the application of the tympanometry and stapedial acoustic reflex test using probe tones of 220/226 Hz, 660/678 Hz, and 1 kHz to young infants (0 to 6 months). Although high-frequency (1 kHz) tympanometry (HFT) has become the standard of practice in pediatric clinics around the globe, the use of stapedial acoustic reflex test with young infants is just emerging. This overview of the literature outlines the development and clinical utility of the HFT to young infants, having acknowledged the inadequacies of traditional tympanometry and acoustic stapedial reflex techniques using low-frequency probe tones. In particular, this chapter updates current research findings on the HFT and stapedial acoustic reflex test, indicating that more research is necessary to advance our understanding of middle ear dynamics in young infants.

TYMPANOMETRY IN YOUNG INFANTS USING LOW-FREQUENCY PROBE TONES

Tympanometric Results from Early Studies

Tympanometry has been used with young infants since the early 1970s (Brooks, 1971). In early studies, conventional tympanometry with a single low-frequency panometry with a single low-frequency

17

probe tone of 220 or 226 Hz was used by many investigators to test the middle ear function of young infants (Bennett, 1975; Groothuis, Altemeier, Wright, & Sell, 1978; Himelfarb, Popelka, & Shanon, 1979; Keith, 1973; Keith & Bench, 1978; Margolis & Popelka, 1975; Margolis & Smith, 1977; Paradise, Smith, & Bluestone, 1976; Pestalozza & Cusmano, 1980; Poulsen & Tos, 1978; Schwartz & Schwartz, 1980; Shurin, Pelton, & Finkelstein, 1977; Shurin, Pelton, & Klein, 1976). Results from these studies indicate that the use of conventional tympanometry with a probe tone of 226 Hz with young infants has been found to be problematic. The test findings were unpredictable and not consistent with the medical diagnoses.

First, researchers often obtained normal single-peaked Type A tympanograms (Jerger, 1970; Liden, 1969) in infants with confirmed middle ear effusion (MEE). For instance, Paradise et al. (1976) were one of the first groups of researchers to cast doubt on the efficacy of conventional tympanometry for this population when they found that about 40% of infants aged less than 6 months with confirmed MEE, based on pneumatic otoscopy and myringotomy findings, exhibited normal tympanograms. This finding is confirmed by Pestalozza and Cusmano (1980) and Schwartz and Schwartz (1980), who found that normal Type A tympanograms were present in 20 to 94% of ears with confirmed MEE. Clearly, this false negative rate is too high to warrant its clinical application for this age group.

Second, researchers found that the use of a low-frequency (220/226 Hz) probe tone can produce flat (Type B) tympanograms in infants with normal healthy ears. For example, Groothius et al. (1978) conducted a longitudinal study to determine the accuracy of tympanometry in predicting the evolution and resolution of acute otitis media (OM) in 71 normal infants aged 4 weeks to 17 months. They found that 93% of infants with normal otoscopic findings had Type B tympanograms. In a longitudinal study of 210 children during the first 2 years of life, Wright, McConnell, Thompson, Vaughn, and Sell (1985) reported that flat tympanogram were found in 37% of young infants, who had normal pneumatic otoscopy results. In essence, the findings from both studies indicate an alarming false positive rate that prohibited conventional tympanometry to be used with young infants.

Last, the use of conventional tympanometry in this age group also resulted in a high proportion of complex or multipeaked tympanograms. For instance, Keith (1973) found that 18% of double-peaked tympanograms were recorded when 220-Hz tympanometry was used to test the middle ear function of 40 neonates aged 36 to 151 hours. In other studies, between 30 and 85% of neonates were reported to have notched or double-peaked tympanograms when tested with conventional tympanometry (Bennett, 1975; Himelfarb et al., 1979; Kei, Allison-Levrick, Dockray, Harrys, Kirkegard, Wong, et al., 2003; Sprague, Wiley, & Goldstein, 1985). These complex tympanograms did not fit in any category of either the Liden or Jerger scheme (Jerger, 1970; Liden, 1969) or the Vanhuyse model (Vanhuyse, Creten,

& Van Camp, 1975). Hence, these complex or multipeaked tympanograms render interpretation of results difficult and, undoubtedly, susceptible to errors.

The erroneous tympanometric findings obtained with low-frequency probe tones have been speculated to result from anatomical differences between the ears of an infant and adult. Although the inner two-thirds of an adult's ear canal wall are surrounded by bone, a young infant's ear canal is cartilaginous (see Chapter 1 for details). The external ear canal of an infant consists of a thin, soft layer of cartilage, resulting in a highly compliant ear canal in response to pressure variations inside the ear canal. Hence, pressurizing the neonatal ear canal during tympanometry may cause distension of the incompletely ossified ear canal walls (Keith, 1975; Paradise et al., 1976). Keith (1975) and Paradise et al. (1976) speculated that movement of the ear canal wall may influence the tympanometric results. In contrast, Holte, Cavanaugh, and Margolis (1990) found no significant associations between ear canal movement and the complexity of the tympanogram shapes. Thus, the exact influence of infant's compliant external ear canal on the conventional tympanometry findings remains unclear.

The anatomical and developmental changes in the middle ear of young infants may contribute to the difference in tympanometric findings between young infants and adults (Holte, Margolis, & Cavanaugh, 1991; Keefe, Bulen, Arehart, & Burns, 1993; Keefe & Levi, 1996; McKinley, Grose, & Roush, 1997; Meyer, Jardine, & Deverson, 1997). The

changes include an increase in size of the middle ear cavity and mastoid; a decrease in the overall mass of the middle ear due to the loss of mesenchyme and changes in bone density; ossicular joint tightening; lesser coupling between the stapes and the annular ligament; fusion of the tympanic ring; and a change in tympanic membrane orientation and its flexibility (Eby & Nadol, 1986; Jaffe, Hurtado, & Hurtado, 1970; Keith, 1975; Mclellan & Webb, 1957; Saunders, Kaltenbach, & Relkin, 1983).

The middle ear of a young infant is dominated more by mass than stiffness elements when compared to that of an adult (Himelfarb et al., 1979; Holte et al., 1991; Hunter & Margolis, 1992; McKinley et al., 1997; Meyer et al., 1997). Evidence is provided by Himelfarb et al. (1979) who found that the reactance component measured in healthy neonates using low-frequency probe tone was always positive and smaller than the resistance component, suggesting a mass-dominated middle ear system in neonates. Furthermore, Holte et al. (1991) found an increase in admittance phase angle with age in 23 infants aged from 0 to 4 months, indicating large mass susceptance at birth which diminishes with age up to 4 months. The transition between mass-dominance to stiffness-dominance in an infant's middle ear system is expected to be complete by 7 to 8 months, when conventional tympanometry may be applied successfully (Alaerts, Luts, & Wouters, 2007).

The pattern of tympanometric results in infants is influenced by the resonance frequency of the middle ear. This resonance frequency is the frequency at which sound of this frequency is enhanced in the middle ear. Meyer et al. (1997) found that the middle ear resonance frequency of an infant increases with age, with the resonance frequency being less than 500 Hz at 14 weeks of age. Recently, Kei, Mazlan, Seshimo, and Wada (2010) estimated the mean resonance frequency in 21 full-term neonates, aged between 1 and 4 days, to be 306.7 Hz (SD = 41.2 Hz). When the resonance frequency of the middle ear of a neonate approaches 226 Hz (the frequency of the probe tone), double- or multipeaked pattern will occur (Kei et al., 2003). Kei et al. (2003) found that 47.5% of 122 healthy newborn infants showed double-peaked tympanograms when a 226-Hz probe tone was used. This finding is in keeping with the findings in earlier studies that a high proportion of young infants exhibited complex notching patterns using the 226-Hz tympanometry (Hirsch, Margolis, & Rykken, 1992; Holte et al., 1991; Keith, 1975; McKinley et al., 1997; Meyer et al., 1997; Sprague et al., 1985; Williams, Purdy, & Barber, 1995). However, the occurrence of multipeaked tympanometric patterns in infants can be reduced if a high probe-tone frequency such as 1 kHz is utilized (Kei et al., 2003).

A possible confounding factor affecting the interpretation of tympanometric findings is associated with the way the admittance of the middle ear is calculated. In conventional tympanometry, the mobility of the eardrum is usually determined by estimating the peak compensated static admittance (commonly known as static admittance), which is calculated by subtracting the admittance of

the ear canal from the uncompensated peak admittance. The calculation of the static admittance rests on the assumption that both the ear canal and the middle ear act as a pure stiffness (compliance) system, with an admittance phase angle of 90° (Shanks & Lily, 1981). In other words, the subtraction of the two vector quantities representing the peak admittance (usually measured at the tympanometric peak pressure or 0 daPa) and ear canal admittance (usually measured at 200 daPa) is accurate only if they are aligned along the same direction. However, this assumption is invalid for neonates who do not have a stiffness-dominated middle ear system. This claim is supported by Kei, Mazlan, Hickson, Gavranich, and Linning (2007) who found that the phase angles of the admittance vectors for a neonate were 67°, 43°, and 40° at ear canal pressure of 200, 0, and −400 daPa, respectively. Hence, the mathematical principles underlying 226 Hz tympanometric measurements, which apply successfully to the adults, are not applicable to neonates.

Tympanometry in Young Infants Using Probe Tones of 660/678 Hz

Having realized the limitations of conventional tympanometry, investigators attempted to use a higher probe tone frequency such as 660/678 Hz for measuring the middle ear function in neonates (Himelfarb et al., 1979; Marchant, McMillan, Shurin, Johnson, Turczyk, Feinstein, et al., 1986; Shurin et al., 1977; Sprague et al., 1985; Sutton, Gleadle, & Rowe, 1996). They were able to get more accurate diagnosis of MEE using the 660/678 Hz than the traditional 220/226-Hz probe tone. For example, Shurin and colleagues (1977) evaluated the diagnostic value of 220 and 660 Hz tympanometry in detecting MEE in 91 children ranging in age from 2 months to 12 years old. They demonstrated better separation between normal ears and ears with MEE utilizing 660 Hz than 220 Hz tympanometry. Marchant et al. (1986) demonstrated good agreement between otoscopy, 660-Hz probe tone tympanometry, and ipsilateral acoustic reflex thresholds (Kappa coefficient = 0.82 to 0.86) in infants younger than 5 months of age. Sutton et al. (1996), after examining the middle ears of 84 special care nursery neonates, concluded that 678-Hz tympanometry was a useful indicator of middle ear status in this special population.

Despite promising results using 660/678-Hz tympanometry in the young infant population, the presence of multipeaked tympanograms impedes its clinical utility. For instance, McKinley et al. (1997) found multipeaked tympanograms in 18% of 55 healthy neonates using 678-Hz tympanometry. In another study, 85% of tympanograms recorded by Himelfarb et al. (1979) were multipeaked tympanograms. The authors proposed that the high compliance of an infant's external ear canal wall might have contributed to the irregularities of 678-Hz tympanograms. This claim is substantiated by the work of Keefe et al. (1993), who measured energy acoustic impedance, acoustic admittance and reflection coefficients using stimuli with frequencies from 125 to 10,700 Hz in full-term infants aged 1 to 24 months. They found that the transmission of sounds between 220 and 660 Hz into the middle ear was not efficient due to possible vibration and resonance of the ear canal wall. From this finding, they concluded that probe tone frequencies between 220 and 660 Hz were the worst possible range to use in infants. In addition, they also demonstrated that sounds with frequencies between 1000 and 4000 Hz were most efficiently transmitted into the middle ear, indicating that stimuli with this frequency range should be used with young infants. Hence, they recommended higher probe tones, above 660 Hz, for the assessment of middle ear function in young infants.

HIGH-FREQUENCY (1 KHZ) TYMPANOMETRY IN YOUNG INFANTS

For the last two decades, a few pilot studies using multifrequency tympanometry have been conducted to investigate the feasibility of using 1-kHz tympanometry (also known as high-frequency tympanometry [HFT]) to detect MEE in young infants. For instance, Williams et al. (1995) obtained tympanometry findings from 26 infants less than 4 months of age using three different probe tones (226, 678, and 1000 Hz). They compared the tympanometric outcomes with otomicroscopy and pneumatic otoscopy results taken as the gold standard and found that the HFT provided the best agreement with the gold standard.

Rhodes, Margolis, Hirsch, and Napp (1999) tested 87 neonatal intensive care unit (NICU) babies and found that 30 to 67% of babies who failed the 226 and 678-Hz tympanometry actually passed a series of electrophysiological tests including otoacoustic emissions (OAEs) and the auditory brainstem response (ABR) test. In their study sample, they found three ears that failed the HFT also failed the OAEs and ABR tests. They concluded that the HFT was more sensitive to middle ear dysfunction than either the 226- or 678-Hz tympanometry. In a longitudinal case study, Meyer et al. (1997) utilized both 226-Hz and 1-kHz probe-tone frequencies to record tympanometric changes in a child from 2 weeks to 6.5 months of age. They found that the HFT provided better diagnostic sensitivity to middle ear dysfunction than conventional tympanometry. This notion was supported by the presence of a flat 1-kHz tympanogram along with a normal 226-Hz tympanogram in the infant with confirmed middle ear pathology. In summary, the findings from these pilot investigations indicated the usefulness of the HFT in identifying middle ear dysfunction in young infants. These pilot studies sparked further systematic investigations into the utility of the HFT with young infants, as recommended by Purdy and Williams (2000).

The amount of research on HFT has been increasing since 2003 (Alaerts et al., 2007; Baldwin, 2006; Calandruccio, Fitzgerald, & Prieve, 2006; Kei et al., 2003; Margolis, Bass-Ringdahl, Hanks, Holte, & Zapala, 2003; Mazlan, Kei, Hickson, Gavranich, & Linning, 2009; Mazlan, Kei, Hickson, Stapleton, Grant, Lim, Gavranich, et al., 2007; Swanepoel,

Werner, Hugo, Louw, Owen, & Swanepoel, 2007). Research, to date, has indicated two schools of thought for interpreting HFT findings in neonates. The first method of interpretation examines the shape or pattern of tympanograms. Although the presence of a positive peak or notching in a tympanogram is regarded as normal, a flat tympanogram indicates the possibility of middle ear dysfunction (Baldwin, 2006; Margolis et al., 2003; Swanepoel et al., 2007). Besides the simple visual admittance classification method, the Vanhuyse model (Vanhuyse et al., 1975) has also been used to categorize the HFT tympanograms according to their shapes (Alaerts et al., 2007; Calandruccio et al., 2006). Specifically, the tympanograms were grouped into either a 1B1G or 3B1G pattern. Using this method, Calandruccio et al. (2006) and Alaerts et al. (2007) found that the Vanhuyse model was adequate for classifying the majority of their HFT results. However, Alaerts et al. (2007) did not recommend its application for clinical purposes because of the complexity in interpreting HFT data for infants less than 3 months of age.

The other method for interpreting HFT findings examines not only the tympanometric contour, but it also inspects some quantitative measures of the tympanogram. These measures include tympanometric peak pressure (TPP), tympanometric width (TW), admittance at +200 daPa (Y_{200}), uncompensated peak admittance (Y_{peak}), peak baseline compensated admittance at +200 daPa (Y_{BC200}), peak baseline compensated admittance at −400 daPa (Y_{BC-400}), and component compensated admittance at

+200 daPa (Y_{CC200}). Researchers have established normative HFT data for newborns and young infants (Alaerts et al., 2007; Calandruccio et al., 2006; Kei et al., 2003; Margolis et al., 2003; Mazlan, Kei, Hickson, Gavranich, et al., 2009; Swanepoel et al., 2007). They recommended relevant cutoff values for some parameters, such as Y_{peak}, Y_{BC200}, Y_{BC-400}, and Y_{CC200}, for use in identifying middle ear dysfunction in young infants. The utility of normative data and criterion cutoff values of some of these parameters in assessing middle ear function in young infants is discussed in Chapter 3.

Test-Retest Reliability of the HFT

In view of the clinical utility of the HFT in assessing middle ear function in young infants, there is a need to evaluate the reliability of the HFT as a clinical tool. In this regard, test-retest reliability is often measured. A clinical procedure is considered reliable if it produces the same results across repeated testing of the same subject under identical conditions. If good test-retest reliability is established, a significant change in the measurements when compared to the baseline results indicates functional changes rather than measurement errors or artifacts (Ruscetta, Palmer, Durrant, Grayhack, & Ryan, 2005). Despite the increasing popularity of HFT in clinical applications, studies on the test-retest reliability of the HFT are scarce.

Kei et al. (2007) investigated the test-retest reliability of the baseline and component compensated static admittances, compensated for ear canal effects at 200 daPa and −400 daPa. They tested 36 neonates twice within the same test session and found no difference in mean static admittance values across the test and retest conditions. Furthermore, they obtained correlation coefficients of 0.89 and 0.92 for the Y_{BC200} and Y_{CC200} (baseline and component compensated static admittances, compensated for ear canal effects at 200 daPa), respectively. However, the correlation coefficient for the baseline compensated static admittance, compensated for ear canal effects at −400 daPa, was 0.58. This pilot study, based on a small sample size, did not report on the test-retest reliability of other HFT parameters such as the tympanometric peak pressure, admittance at +200 daPa, and uncompensated peak admittance.

The test-retest reliability of an instrument may also be affected by subject characteristics. Although newborn babies are usually tested in a sleep or quiet state, older babies such as 6-week-old infants are more active and restless (Mazlan et al., 2007). There might also be differences in anatomical and acoustical properties of the auditory system between two age groups, which might affect the test-retest reliability of the measurements. Mazlan, Kei, Hickson, Gavranich, and Linning (2010) studied the test-retest reliability of HFT in two groups of healthy young infants. A total of 273 newborn babies were assessed twice (Test 1 and Test 2) on the same day, followed by two more assessments (Test 3 and Test 4) for 118 babies who were assessed 6 weeks later. Five HFT measures including the TPP, Y_{200}, Y, Y_{BC200}, and Y_{CC200} were assessed for test-retest reliability. The results showed no significant differences in mean values of the HFT results between the test and retest conditions for the newborn (Test 1/Test 2) and 6-week-old babies (Test 3/Test 4). High reliability for all HFT measures was found for both age groups, as judged by the high intra-correlation coefficients of between 0.75 and 0.95, as shown in Table 2–1. In general, the 6-week-old infants had slightly higher correlation coefficients than the neonates.

To measure the normal variability of the HFT measures, the differences in HFT findings across test and retest conditions may be expressed in absolute (always positive) values. These absolute differences reflect the changes between two measurements regardless of the direction of change. Table 2–2 shows the mean, SD, and 95th percentiles of the differences of the HFT parameters for the newborn and 6-week-old infants.

Normal variability of HFT measures is assumed if the test-retest difference in measurements falls below the 95th percentile value. This criterion of normal variability may be helpful in determining if a change in HFT results between two tests was due to normal test-retest variability or a genuine change in middle ear function due to a medical condition or equipment failure (e.g., an eartip being blocked or a drift in calibration of the equipment).

EFFECT OF AGE ON TYMPANOMETRIC FINDINGS

Little is known about the effect of age on HFT results in young infants. Preliminary tympanometric findings using a probe tone of 900 Hz indicate that the

TABLE 2–1. Intracorrelation Coefficient (ICC) and Statistical Significance (*p*) for the HFT Measures Across Test and Retest Conditions, Obtained from 273 Neonates and 118 6-Week-Old Infants

Test Parameter	ICC Neonates	ICC 6-Week-Old Infants
Tympanometric Peak Pressure, TPP	0.75	0.92
Admittance at +200 daPa, Y_{200}	0.86	0.90
Uncompensated peak admittance, Y	0.90	0.95
Magnitude compensated static admittance, Y_{MC}	0.89	0.86
Component compensated static admittance, Y_{CC}	0.86	0.91

Note: All ICCs were significant, *p* <0.0001.

TABLE 2–2. Test-Retest Differences Expressed in Absolute (always positive) Values for 273 Newborns and 118 6-Week-Old Babies

HFT parameter	Age Group	Mean	SD	95th percentile
Tympanometric Peak Pressure, TPP (daPa)	Newborn	22.8	31.9	66.7
	6-weeks	16.9	18.6	64.2
Admittance at +200 daPa, Y_{200} (mmho)	Newborn	0.13	0.15	0.35
	6-weeks	0.12	0.11	0.36
Uncompensated peak admittance, Y (mmho)	Newborn	0.16	0.22	0.45
	6-weeks	0.16	0.15	0.44
Baseline compensated static admittance at 200 daPa, Y_{BC200} (mmho)	Newborn	0.11	0.11	0.36
	6-weeks	0.17	0.18	0.60
Component compensated static admittance at 200 daPa, Y_{CC200} (mmho)	Newborn	0.14	0.21	0.44
	6-weeks	0.17	0.18	0.52

static admittance obtained from infants aged from 0 to 4 months increases with age (Holte et al., 1991). These findings suggest that tympanometric findings at high probe-tone frequencies increase with age in the early months of life. Keefe et al. (1993) suggest that maturational changes in the anatomy and physiology of the middle ear system of an infant would affect tympanometry results during the first two years of life.

Despite the acknowledgment of this fast developing period, there is limited research to investigate if there are differences in the tympanometric data obtained from infants at various developmental stages. To date, the effect of maturational changes on HFT results has been investigated in four studies. In the first study, Prieve, Chasmawala, and Jackson (2005) performed tympa-nometry in a group of 22 infants from 4 weeks to 2 years of age using probe frequencies of 226, 400, 630, and 1000 Hz. In this study, 22 normally hearing adults served as controls. Their findings indicated that the middle ear admittance value increased with increasing age at all probe frequencies, with infants having lower static admittance values than adults. In the second study, Calandruccio et al. (2006) conducted a longitudinal investigation of static admittance values of 33 infants aged 4 weeks to 2 years. Using a 1-kHz probe tone, the authors found that infants aged 4 to 19 weeks had significantly lower middle ear admittance values than those aged 6 months to 2 years. In the third study, Swanepoel et al. (2007) tested 143 healthy neonates aged between 1 and 28 days using the HFT. They found that the median value of the uncompensated peak admittance (Y_{peak}) for males increased from 2.18 mmho for newborns to 2.30 mmho for infants aged 2 to 4 weeks, whereas for females, Y_{peak} increased from 1.8 to 2.4 mmho for the corresponding period. The TPP ranged from 5 to −15 daPa and there was no apparent change in TPP during this period. In the fourth study, Mazlan et al. (2007) compared the HFT parameters obtained from healthy neonates at birth and 6 weeks using a longitudinal design. Newborns were found to exhibit significantly smaller mean values in Y_{200} (1.1 vs. 1.3 mmho), Y_{peak} (1.9 vs. 2.4 mmho), and Y_{BC200} (0.8 vs. 1.0 mmho) than those obtained 6 weeks later. No significant differences in mean TPPs occurred during this 6-week period. In summary, the findings from the above four studies support the proposition that developmental changes in HFT findings occur during the infant's first few months of life. These findings indicate the importance of having a separate normative data set for different age groups.

VALIDATION OF HFT IN DETECTING MIDDLE EAR DYSFUNCTION IN NEONATES

Validation of the HFT results requires a comparison of HFT findings with a gold standard. However, surgical findings in neonates are rarely available, and otoscopic examination in their tiny ears is often difficult (Rhodes et al., 1999). Moreover, pneumatic otoscopy appears to be unreliable. For instance, Shurin et al. (1976) reported that five out of 10 newborn ears diagnosed with MEE by otoscopy were found to have normal or dry ear on tympanocentesis. In a study of MEE in infants using auditory brainstem response (ABR), transient evoked otoacoustic emissions (TEOAEs), and pneumatic otoscopy, Doyle, Burggraaff, Fujikawa, Kim, and Macarthur (1997) reported that 9% of examined ears had presumed MEE, based on reduced tympanic membrane mobility observed from pneumatic otoscopy. Of those ears with reduced mobility, half of them passed the ABR screening test, and about one-third passed the TEOAE screen, suggesting that the use of pneumatic otoscopy in newborn babies can result in incorrect diagnosis.

In the absence of a realistic gold standard for identifying MEE in neonates, the use of other tests of auditory function, such as TEOAEs have been employed to validate the HFT results (e.g., Kei et al., 2003; Margolis et al., 2003). Because TEOAEs require efficient transmission of sound to and from cochlea, the presence of TEOAEs provides some level of assurance of normal middle ear function. However, TEOAEs alone are not perfect as a gold standard because TEOAEs can be recorded in some ears with middle ear dysfunction (Driscoll, Kei, & McPherson, 2000; Thornton, Kimm, Kennedy, & Cafarelli-Dees, 1993). A possible method to be used in conjunction with the HFT test for identifying middle ear dysfunction in young infants is the incorporation of acoustic stapedial reflex (ASR) testing in the test battery (Hirsch et al., 1992; Purdy & Williams, 2000). The ASR test has been found to be sensitive to middle ear disorders (Jerger, Burney, Mauldin, & Crump, 1974). Perhaps, the use of a battery of tests including TEOAE, HFT, and ASR tests may be an accurate measure for detecting middle ear dysfunction in young infants. Chapter 3 gives an account of the application of HFT to young infants.

ACOUSTIC STAPEDIAL REFLEX IN YOUNG INFANTS

Early studies on the use of ASR (using low probe-tone frequencies of 220 and 226 Hz) with healthy young infants reported raised or absent reflexes (Abahazi & Greenberg, 1977; Bennett, 1975; Keith, 1973; Keith & Bench, 1978; McCandless & Allred, 1978; Stream, Stream, Walker,

& Breningstall, 1978). Table 2–3 provides a summary of the findings from seven studies, showing the percentage presence of ASRs in neonates when reflexes were elicited by tonal or noise activators using a 220/226-Hz probe tone. For instance, Keith (1973) found clear ASR responses to 0.5- and 2-kHz tones at 100 dB HL in only 36% of 40 normal healthy neonates aged 36 to 151 hours after birth. Bennett (1975) reported that only 16% of 98 normal neonates ranging in age from 5 to 218 hours exhibited ASRs using a 226-Hz probe tone. In a later study, Keith and Bench (1978) found neonates to have ASR responses to a 1-kHz tone and noise stimulus in only 5.4% of cases. Except for the Vincent and Gerber (1987) study, the percentage of presence of ASR in normal neonates was low. Overall, the results from these studies indicate that

TABLE 2–3. Summary of Findings from Seven Studies Showing the Percentage Presence of ASRs in Neonates When Reflexes Were Elicited by Tonal or Noise Activators Using a 220/226-Hz Probe Tone

Study	N (ears)	Stimuli	Age	Presence of ASRs (%)
Keith (1973)	40	0.5 & 2 kHz	36–51 hours	36
Bennett (1975)	98	noise	5–218 hours	16
Keith & Bench (1978)	20	1 kHz & noise	18–192 hours	5.4
Himelfarb et al. (1978)	21	0.5–4 kHz & BBN*	8–96 hours	17–88
McMillan et al. (1985)	47	0.5–4 kHz	10–118 hours	20–24
Sprague et al. (1985)	53	BBN and 1 kHz	24–105 hours	80
Vincent & Gerber (1987)	40	0.5–4 kHz & BBN	24–28 hours	100

*BBN stands for broadband noise.

ASRs are not consistently present in young infants when a low-frequency probe tone is used.

The unsuccessful recording of ASRs in the neonatal population using a low-frequency probe tone has led researchers to investigate the use of probe tone frequencies higher than 226 Hz. Table 2–4 provides a summary of findings from seven studies showing the percentage presence of ASRs in neonates when reflexes were elicited by tonal or noise activators using a 660/678-Hz probe tone. Although the percentage of presence of ASR was generally higher than that using a 220/226-Hz probe tone, the target of eliciting ASRs in all healthy neonates was not consistently achieved.

According to Weatherby and Bennett (1980), the difficulty of eliciting ASRs using a low-frequency probe tone is due to the mismatch in acoustic impedance between tympanic membrane and the middle ear. The authors found that the tympanic membrane in a neonate has low acoustic impedance at low-frequency probe tones (e.g., 220/226 Hz), whereas the middle ear system has high acoustic impedance. This mismatch in impedance makes it difficult to detect the small changes in middle ear impedance associated with ASR activation. Therefore, the use of a probe tone with low frequency is not recommended when measuring ASR in the neonatal population.

Of particular importance is the finding from Weatherby and Bennett (1980) that the presence of ASR in neonates does not only depend on the stimulus type and intensity, but it also depends on the frequency of the probe tone. In

TABLE 2–4. Summary of Findings from Seven Studies Showing the Percentage Presence of ASRs in Neonates When Reflexes Were Elicited by Tonal or Noise Activators Using a 660/678-Hz Probe Tone

Study	N (ears)	Stimuli	Age	Presence of ASRs (%)
Margolis & Popelka (1975)	20	0.5–4 kHz	55–132 days	80
McCandless & Allred (1978)	53	0.5–4 kHz	4–51 hours	89
Weatherby & Bennett (1980)	30	*BBN	18–192 hrs	93.3
Sprague et al. (1985)	53	BBN and 1 kHz	24–105 hours	74–81
Marchant et al. (1986)	86	1 kHz	2–18 weeks	80
Geddes (1987)	45	BBN	1–120 hours	83.3
Sutton et al. (1996)	168	2 kHz	3–134 hrs	41.7

*BBN stands for broadband noise.

a study sample of 44 neonates aged between 10 and 169 hours, they were able to elicit ASR when the frequency of the probe tone was 800 Hz or higher. They recommended the use of a probe tone frequency within the range of 800 to 1800 Hz for neonatal testing. This is a clinically significant finding that confirms the integrity of the auditory system of healthy neonates to respond to loud sounds. Subsequent studies have supported Weatherby and Bennett's (1980) finding. For example, ASRs were recorded from all 28 healthy neonates, aged 4 to 8 days, using a 1200-Hz probe tone (Bennett & Weatherby, 1982). In another study, Hirsch et al. (1992) measured ASR in 76 babies aged 32 to 56 weeks in the neonatal intensive care unit (NICU) using a probe tone frequency of 800 Hz with a 2-kHz tone and noise as stimuli. ASRs were present in 61% (91/149) of ears tested. Similar results were obtained by Rhodes and colleagues (1999), who found that 87% of 173 NICU babies showed the presence of ASR when a 1-kHz probe tone and an activating stimulus of 2 kHz were used. In essence, these studies indicate that ASRs are consistently present in young infants when a high-frequency probe tone is used.

ASR with a Probe Tone of 1 kHz in Young Infants: Recent Studies

Despite early studies showing that ASR with a probe tone of 1 kHz can be reliably obtained from healthy neonates, no further development of this test has been made until recently. The imple-mentation of universal newborn hearing screening programs around the world has provided a platform for further investigation into the use of ASR with young infants. Absence of ASR or raised acoustic stapedial reflex thresholds (ASRTs) may indicate the possibility of middle ear dysfunction, severe cochlear impairment, or retrocochlear lesion such as auditory neuropathy/dys-synchrony (also known as auditory neuropathy spectrum disorder) in the test ear (Berlin, Hood, Morlet, Wilensky, Li, Mattingly, et al., 2010; Berlin, Hood, Morlet, Wilensky, St. John, Montgomery, et al., 2005; Gelfand, 2002; Margolis & Levine, 1991). Given these potential clinical applications, the ASR can play an important role in the diagnosis of auditory dysfunction in young infants. To date, a few studies have been conducted to investigate the feasibility of obtaining ASR and the prevalence of ASR in young infants.

Swanepoel and colleagues (2007) investigated the use of ASR testing in conjunction with the HFT. In this study, ipsilateral ASRs were recorded following tympanometry at the tympanometric peak pressure at which maximum admittance occurred. They recorded ASRTs from 143 neonates aged 0 to 4 weeks using a 1-kHz probe tone and a 1-kHz pure-tone stimulus. The ASRT was defined as the lowest intensity level of the stimulus when a change of admittance of at least 0.02 mmho occurred. Based on this criterion, they found that 94% of ears exhibited ASRs with a mean threshold of 93 dB HL. This level is greater than 82 to 85 dB HL obtained by Sprague et al. (1985) and Vincent and Gerber (1987) for a stimulus tone of 1 kHz with low-frequency probe tones (220 Hz and 660 Hz). The high mean ASRT obtained by Swanepoel et al. (2007) may be due to the probe and stimulating tones having the same frequency so that the stimulus tone intensity had to be greater than that of the probe tone to elicit an ASR.

To avoid possible interactions of the stimulus tone with the probe tone, Mazlan and colleagues (2007) used a 2-kHz tone and broadband noise (BBN) to elicit ASRs from healthy newborns using a probe tone of 1 kHz. In their study, they were successful in eliciting ASRs from all 42 participants who passed both the TEOAE and automated ABR (AABR) tests. One randomly selected ear from each neonate was tested. The ASR test was performed after a normal tympanogram was obtained from the neonate. The ASRTs for both stimuli were determined using an auto threshold search mode of the equipment. In this mode, the device (Madsen Otoflex 100) registered an ASR response when the change in admittance, in either the upward (increase) or downward (decrease) direction, was at least 0.04 mmho. The mean ipsilateral ASR thresholds for the 2-kHz and the broadband activators were 73 dB HL and 59 dB HL, respectively. The mean ASR for the broadband noise may have been overestimated because some neonates were likely to have an ASRT below 50 dB HL. However, the device could not present stimuli below 50 dB HL.

In a follow-up study, Kei (in press) established normative ASR data using the same equipment and test procedure.

Participants were 69 full-term neonates who passed the AABR, TEOAE, and HFT tests. An ASR was considered present when the change in admittance in either direction (increase or decrease) was 0.04 mmho or greater. The increase in admittance may be due to a functional decoupling of the stapes from the cochlea, thereby reducing sound energy to be transferred to the inner ear (Borg, 1968; Moller, 1961). Kei (in press) demonstrated that ASR was present in 98.6% of the 69 neonates when stimulated ipsilaterally by tonal stimuli (0.5, 2, and 4 kHz) or BBN. The mean ASRTs for the 0.5-, 2-, and 4-kHz tones were 81.6 dB HL (SD = 7.9 dB), 71.3 dB HL (SD = 7.9), and 65.4 dB HL (SD = 8.7 dB), respectively. Further analysis reviewed that the mean ASRT for 0.5 kHz was significantly greater than that for 2 kHz, which in turn was significantly greater than that for 4 kHz. The mean ASRT for the BBN was estimated to be smaller than 57.2 dB HL, given the limitation of the equipment. Interestingly, the upward reflex pattern was found in 32.4% (22/68), 20.6% (14/68), 23.5% (16/68), and 11.8% (8/68) of ears stimulated by 0.5 kHz, 2 kHz, 4 kHz, and BBN, respectively. The 95th percentiles of the ASRT were 95, 85, 80, and 75 dB HL for 0.5, 2, 4 kHz, and BBN, respectively. These ASRT levels represent the upper limit of the normative data, beyond which ASR findings are considered abnormal. Further research to establish contralateral ASRT normative data may be necessary in the near future if a comprehensive evaluation of ASR in young infants is warranted.

Test-Retest Reliability of the ASR Test

For the ASR test (with a probe tone of 1 kHz) to be widely accepted as a clinical tool, the results should be repeatable or the test-retest difference in ASRT be within limits of normal variability. Three studies investigating the test-retest reliability of the ASR test for young infants have been published, to date.

In the first study, Mazlan, Kei, and Hickson (2009) evaluated the test-retest reliability of ipsilateral ASRT in 219 healthy neonates aged between 1 and 8 days. Neonates included in the study had to pass a series of tests, including the AABR, TEOAE, and HFT tests, for both the test and retest conditions. One randomly selected ear from each neonate was tested. As a result of the inclusion criteria, only 194 and 123 ears were included in the test-retest reliability analysis for the 2-kHz tone and BBN stimuli, respectively. Following the HFT test, the ASRTs for both stimuli were determined using an auto threshold search mode of the equipment as described in the Mazlan et al.

(2007) study. An ASR response was considered when the change in admittance, in either the upward (increase) or downward (decrease) direction, was at least 0.04 mmho. On completion of the first test, the probe was removed from the ear, a new seal attained and the procedures for HFT and ASR tests repeated to obtain a second set of ASR findings.

Table 2–5 shows the descriptive statistics of the ASRTs for the 2-kHz pure tone and BBN stimuli. As shown in Table 2–5, there is no significant difference in mean ASRTs between the test and retest conditions for both stimuli.

The test-retest reliability of the ASR test was also assessed by calculating the intra-correlation coefficients (ICCs) of the ASRTs across the test-retest conditions. The results showed that the test and retest conditions are highly correlated with ICCs of 0.83 and 0.76 for the 2-kHz tone and BBN, respectively.

In the second study conducted by Mazlan, Kei, Hickson, Curtain, et al. (2009), the test-retest reliability of ASRT was measured in a group of 6-week-old infants who passed the AABR, TEOAE, and HFT tests. Ipsilateral ASRTs for a

TABLE 2–5. Ipsilateral Acoustic Stapedial Reflex Thresholds (ASRTs) Elicited by Broadband Noise (BBN) and 2-kHz Pure-Tone Stimuli from Newborn Babies in the Test and Retest Conditions

| Stimulus | N (ears) | Test Condition ASRTs (dB HL) | | Retest Condition ASRTs (dB HL) | |
		Mean ± SD	90% range	Mean ± SD	90% range
BBN	123	64.9 ± 7.8	55.0–80.0	64.4 ± 7.9	55.0–75.0
2-kHz tone	194	76.2 ± 7.9	65.0–90.0	76.0 ± 8.1	65.0–90.0

2 kHz pure tone and broadband noise were recorded from 70 infants using a Madsen Otoflex device with a probe tone of 1 kHz. The mean ASRTs obtained in the first test were 80.9 and 67.3 dB HL for the 2-kHz tone and broadband noise, respectively. After completion of the first test, the probe was removed from the ear, a new seal attained and the procedure repeated. The results for the retest condition did not differ significantly from those of the first test. The ASR test also showed high test-retest reliability as demonstrated by intracorrelation coefficients across the test-retest conditions of 0.78 for both stimuli.

The third study was an extension of the Mazlan, Kei, and Hickson (2009) study. In addition to the use of 2 kHz and BBN as stimuli, Kei (in press) investigated the test-retest reliability of ASRT for two more stimuli (0.5- and 4-kHz tones). The results showed no significant difference in mean ASRT between the test and retest conditions regardless of the stimuli used. The percentage of measurements showing normal variability (within ±10 dB) across test and retest conditions were in excess of 90% for all stimuli. The intracorrelation coefficients between test and retest findings were 0.66, 0.78, 0.74, and 0.63 for the 0.5, 2, 4 kHz, and BBN, respectively.

In summary, the three studies provided evidence that the ASRT for the tonal and BBN stimuli is repeatable across the test and retest conditions. The ASR test can be used in a battery of tests to diagnose hearing impairment in young infants. Chapter 4 provides an account of the clinical application of the ASR test to young infants.

OTHER STRATEGIES TO ASSESS THE MIDDLE EAR FUNCTION OF YOUNG INFANTS

Middle ear disorder in young infants is often missed unless an effective test procedure for middle ear function is in place. In addition to the HFT and ASR tests, three other techniques have been trialed to assess the middle ear function of neonates: the multifrequency tympanometry, the sweep frequency impedance, and the wideband acoustic transfer functions.

Multifrequency tympanometry enables tympanometry to be performed at various probe tone frequencies including frequencies close to 1 kHz. The multifrequency technique measures the conductance and susceptance of a middle ear system at various probe-tone frequencies. Using this technique, it is possible to measure the resonance frequency of the middle ear system. As an abnormal middle ear has a characteristic resonance frequency that is different from that of a normal ear, the multifrequency tympanometry has the potential to separate abnormal from normal middle ears in clinical situations. This technique is discussed in detail in Chapter 5.

The sweep frequency impedance (SFI), originally developed by Hiroshi Wada for use with adults, is a variation of the multifrequency technique (Wada, Kobayashi, Suetake, & Tachiki, 1989). The SFI equipment has recently been modified for use with young infants. The SFI measures the intensity level of sound inside the ear canal as a function of the frequency of the sweep tone and applied air pressure. With this technique, it is possible to measure the resonance frequency of the middle ear and the mobility of the eardrum. Pilot studies have been carried out both in Japan and Australia with promising results. Chapter 6 provides an account of the development of the SFI device and its potential application to young infants.

The wideband acoustic transfer functions technique measures the reflectance of sound such as a click or a chirp presented to the ear canal. The wideband acoustic transfer functions for young infants are established to measure how much acoustic energy is transmitted into the middle ear. In ears with abnormal middle ear function, the test results will fall outside the normal limits. With the assistance of the Interacoustics Pty Ltd. in Denmark, the device is available for research purposes. Research in this area is continuing. Chapter 7 introduces the principles of this technique and examines test findings obtained from adults and young infants.

REFERENCES

Abahazi, D. A., & Greenberg, H. J. (1977). Clinical acoustic reflex threshold measurements in infants. *Journal of Speech and Hearing Disorders, 42,* 514–519.

Alaerts, J., Luts, H., & Wouters, J. (2007). Evaluation of middle ear function in young children: Clinical guidelines for the use of 226- and 1000-Hz tympanometry. *Otology and Neurotology, 28,* 727–732.

Baldwin, M. (2006). Choice of probe tone and classification of trace patterns in tympanometry undertaken in early infancy. *International Journal of Audiology, 45,* 417–427.

Bennett, M. J. (1975). Acoustic impedance measurements with the neonates. *British Journal of Audiology, 9,* 117.

Bennett, M. J., & Weatherby, L. A. (1982). Newborn acoustic reflexes to noise and pure-tone signals. *Journal of Speech and Hearing Research, 25,* 383–387.

Berlin, C. I., Hood, L. J., Morlet, T., Wilensky, D., Li, L., Mattingly K. R., . . . Frisch, S. A. (2010). Multi-site diagnosis and management of 260 patients with auditory neuropathy/dys-synchrony (auditory neuropathy spectrum disorder). *International Journal of Audiology, 49,* 30–43.

Berlin, C. I., Hood, L. J., Morlet, T., Wilensky, D., St. John, P., Montgomery, E., & Thibodaux, M. (2005). Absent or elevated middle ear muscle reflexes in the presence of normal otoacoustic emissions: A universal finding in 136 cases of auditory neuropathy/dys-synchrony. *Journal of the American Academy of Audiology, 16,* 546–553.

Borg, E. (1968). A quantitative study of the effect of the acoustic stapedius reflex on sound transmission through the middle ear of man. *Acta Otolaryngologica (Stockholm), 66,* 461.

Brooks, D. N. (1971). A new approach to identification audiometry. *Audiology, 10,* 334-339.

Calandruccio, L., Fitzgerald, T. S., & Prieve, B. A. (2006). Normative multifrequency tympanometry in infants and toddlers. *Journal of the American Academy of Audiology 17,* 470–480.

Doyle, K., Burggraaff, B., Fujikawa, S., Kim, J., & Macarthur, C. (1997). Neonatal hearing screening with otoscopy, auditory brain stem response, and otoacoustic emissions. *Otolaryngology-Head and Neck Surgery, 116,* 597–603.

Driscoll, C., Kei, J., & McPherson, B. (2000). Transient evoked otoacoustic emissions in six-year-old school children: A normative study. *Scandinavian Audiology*, *29*, 103–110.

Eby, T. L., & Nadol, J. B. (1986). Abnormalities of the neonatal ear: Otoscopic observations, histologic observations, and a model for contamination of the middle ear by cellular contents of amniotic fluid. *Laryngoscope*, *103*, 1–31.

Geddes, N. (1987). Tympanometry and the stapedial reflex in the first five days of life. *International Journal of Pediatric Otorhinolaryngology*, *13*, 293–297.

Gelfand, S. A. (2002). The acoustic reflex. In J. Katz (Ed.), *Handbook of clinical audiology* (5th ed.). New York, NY: Lippincott Williams & Wilkins.

Groothuis, J., Altemeier, W., Wright, P., & Sell, S. (1978). The evolution and resolution of otitis media in infants: Tympanometric findings. In E. Harford, F. Bess, C. Bluestone, & J. Klein (Eds.), *Impedance screening for middle ear disease in children*. New York, NY: Grune and Stratton.

Himelfarb, M. Z., Popelka, G. R., & Shanon, E. (1979). Tympanometry in normal neonates. *Journal of Speech and Hearing Research*, *22*, 179–191.

Hirsch, J. E., Margolis, R. H., & Rykken, J. R. (1992). A comparison of acoustic reflex and auditory brainstem response screening of high-risk infants. *Ear and Hearing*, *13*, 181–186.

Holte, L., Cavanaugh, R., & Margolis, R. H. (1990). Ear canal wall mobility and tympanometric shape in young infants. *Journal of Pediatrics*, *117*, 77–80.

Holte, L., Margolis, R. H., & Cavanaugh, R. (1991). Developmental changes in multifrequency tympanograms. *Audiology 30*, 1–24.

Hunter, L., & Margolis, R. H. (1992). Multifrequency tympanometry: Current clinical application. *American Journal of Audiology*, *1*, 33–43.

Jaffe, B. F., Hurtado, F., & Hurtado, E. (1970). Tympanic membrane mobility in the newborn (with seven months' follow-up). *Laryngoscope*, *80*, 36–48.

Jerger, J. (1970). Clinical experience with impedance audiometry. *Archives of Otolaryngology*, *92*, 311–324.

Jerger, J., Burney, P., Mauldin, L., & Crump, B. (1974). Predicting hearing loss from the acoustic reflex. *Journal of the Speech and Hearing Disorders*, *39*, 11–17.

Keefe, D. H., Bulen, J. C., Arehart, K. H., & Burns, E. M. (1993). Ear-canal impedance and reflection coefficient in human infants and adults. *Journal of the Acoustical Society of America*, *94*, 2617–2638.

Keefe, D. H., & Levi, E. (1996). Maturation of the middle and external ears: Acoustic power-based responses and reflectance tympanometry. *Ear and Hearing*, *17*, 361–373.

Kei, J. (in press). Acoustic stapedial reflexes in healthy neonates: Normative data and test-retest reliability. *Journal of the American Academy of Audiology*.

Kei, J., Allison-Levrick, J., Dockray, J., Harrys, R., Kirkegard, C., Wong, J., . . . Tudehope, D. (2003). High-frequency (1000 Hz) tympanometry in normal neonates. *Journal of the American Academy of Audiology*, *14*, 20–28.

Kei, J., Mazlan, R., Hickson, L., Gavranich, J., & Linning, R. (2007). Measuring middle ear admittance in newborns using 1000-Hz tympanometry: A comparison of methodologies. *Journal of the American Academy of Audiology*, *18*, 739–748.

Kei, J., Mazlan, R., Seshimo, N., & Wada, H. (2010, May). Measuring middle ear resonant frequency in neonates: A preliminary study. *Proceedings of the XIX National Conference of the Audiological Society of Australia, Sydney*. p. 80.

Keith, R. W. (1973). Impedance audiometry with neonates. *Archives of Otolaryngology, 97*, 465.

Keith, R. W. (1975). Middle ear function in neonates. *Archives of Otolaryngology, 101*, 376–379.

Keith, R. W., & Bench, R. J. (1978). Stapedial reflex in neonates. *Scandinavian Audiology, 7*, 187–191.

Liden, G. (1969). The scope and application of current audiometric tests. *Journal of Laryngology and Otology, 83*, 507–520.

Marchant, C. D., McMillan, P. M., Shurin, P. A., Johnson, C. E., Turczyk, R. N., Feinstein, J. C., & Panek, D. M. (1986). Objective diagnosis of otitis media in early infancy by tympanometry and ipsilateral acoustic reflex thresholds. *Journal of Pediatrics, 109*, 590–595.

Margolis, R. H., Bass-Ringdahl, S., Hanks, W. D., Holte, L., & Zapala, D. A. (2003). Tympanometry in newborn infants—1 kHz norms. *Journal of the American Academy of Audiology, 14*, 383–391.

Margolis, R. H., & Levine, S. (1991). Acoustic reflex measures in audiologic evaluation. *Otolaryngology Clinics of North America, 24*, 329–347.

Margolis, R. H., & Popelka, G. R. (1975). Static and dynamic acoustic impedance measurements in infant ears. *Journal of Speech and Hearing Research, 18*, 435–443.

Margolis, R. H., & Smith, P. (1977). Tympanometric asymmetry. *Journal of Speech and Hearing Research, 20*, 437–446.

Mazlan, R., Kei, J., & Hickson, L. (2009). Test-retest reliability of acoustic reflex testing in healthy newborns. *Ear and Hearing, 30*, 295–301.

Mazlan, R., Kei, J., Hickson, L., Curtain, S., Baker, G., Jarman, K., . . . Linning, R. (2009). Test-retest reliability of acoustic reflex test in 6-week-old healthy infants. *Australian and New Zealand Journal of Audiology, 31*, 25–32.

Mazlan, R., Kei, J., Hickson, L., Gavranich, J., & Linning, R. (2009). High-frequency (1000 Hz) tympanometry findings in newborns: Normative data using a component compensated admittance approach. *Australian and New Zealand Journal of Audiology, 31*, 15–24.

Mazlan, R., Kei, J., Hickson, L., Gavranich, J., & Linning, R. (2010). Test-retest reproducibility of the 1000-Hz tympanometry in newborn and 6-week-old healthy infants. *International Journal of Audiology, 49*, 815–822.

Mazlan, R., Kei, J., Hickson, L., Stapleton, C., Grant, S., Lim, S., Gavranich, J., & Linning, R. (2007). High frequency immittance findings: Newborn versus six-week-old infants. *International Journal of Audiology, 46*, 711–717.

McCandless, G., & Allred, P. (1978). Tympanometry and emergence of the acoustic reflex in infants. In E. Harford, F. Bess, C. Bluestone, & J. Klein (Eds.), *Impedance screening for middle ear disease in children*. New York, NY: Grune and Stratton.

McKinley, A. M., Grose, J. H., & Roush, J. (1997). Multifrequency tympanometry and evoked otoacoustic emissions in neonates during the first 24 hours of life. *Journal of the American Academy of Audiology, 8*, 218–223.

Mclellan, M. S., & Webb, C. H. (1957). Ear studies in the newborn infant. *Journal of Pediatrics, 51*, 672–677.

McMillan, P. M., Bennett, M. J., Marchant, C. D., & Shurin, P. A. (1985). Ipsilateral and contralateral acoustic reflexes in neonates. *Ear and Hearing, 6*, 320–324.

Meyer, S. E., Jardine, C. A., & Deverson, W. (1997). Developmental changes in tympanometry: A case study. *British Journal of Audiology, 31*, 189–195.

Moller, A. R. (1961). Bilateral contraction of the tympanic muscles in man. *Annals of*

Otology, Rhinology and Laryngology, 70, 733–752.

Paradise, J. L., Smith, C. G., & Bluestone, C. D. (1976). Tympanometric detection of middle ear effusion in infants and young children. *Pediatrics, 58,* 198–210.

Pestalozza, G., & Cusmano, G. (1980). Evaluation of tympanometry in diagnosis and treatment of otitis media of the newborn and of the infant, *International Journal of Pediatric Otorhinolaryngology, 2,* 73–82.

Poulsen, G., & Tos, M. (1978). Screening tympanometry in newborn infants during the first six months of life. *Scandinavian Audiology, 7,* 159–166.

Prieve, B. A., Chasmawala, S., & Jackson, M. (2005, February 19–24). Development of middle-ear admittance in humans. Association for Research in Otolaryngology. *Abstracts of the ARO Mid-Winter Meeting.* New Orleans, LA, USA. p. 692.

Purdy, S., & Williams, M. J. (2000). High frequency tympanometry: A valid and reliable immittance test protocol for young infants? *New Zealand Audiological Society Bulletin, 10,* 9–24.

Rhodes, M. C., Margolis, R. H., Hirsch, J. E., & Napp, A. P. (1999). Hearing screening in the newborn intensive care nursery: Comparison of methods. *Otolaryngology-Head and Neck Surgery 120,* 799–808.

Ruscetta, M. N., Palmer, C. V., Durrant, J. D., Grayhack, J., & Ryan, C. (2005). Validity, internal consistency, and test/retest reliability of a localization disabilities and handicaps questionnaire. *Journal of the American Academy of Audiology, 16,* 585–595.

Saunders, J. C., Kaltenbach, J. A. & Relkin, E. M. (1983). The structural and functional development of the outer and middle ear. In R. Romand & M. R. Romand (Eds.), *Development of auditory and vestibular systems.* New York, NY: Academic.

Schwartz, D. M., & Schwartz, R. H. (1980). Acoustic immittance finding in acute otitis media. *Annals of Otology, Rhinology and Laryngology, 68,* 211–213.

Shanks, J., & Lily, D. (1981). An evaluation of tympanometric estimates of ear canal volume. *Journal of Speech and Hearing Research, 24,* 557–566.

Shurin, P. A., Pelton, S., & Finkelstein, J. (1977). Tympanometry in the diagnosis of middle ear effusion. *New Zealand Journal of Medicine, 296,* 412–417.

Shurin, P. A., Pelton, S., & Klein, J. (1976). Otitis media in the newborn infant. *Annals of Otology, Rhinology and Laryngology, 85*(Suppl. 25), 216–222.

Sprague, B. H., Wiley, T. L., & Goldstein, R. (1985). Tympanometric and acoustic-reflex studies in neonates. *Journal of Speech and Hearing Research, 28,* 265–272.

Stream, R., Stream, K., Walker, J., & Breningstall, G. (1978). Emerging characteristics of the acoustic reflex in infants. *Otolaryngology, 86,* 628–636.

Sutton, G., Gleadle, P., & Rowe, S. (1996). Tympanometry and otoacoustic emissions in a cohort of special care neonates. *British Journal of Audiology, 30,* 9–17.

Swanepoel, D. W., Werner, S., Hugo, R., Louw, B., Owen, R., & Swanepoel, A. (2007). High-frequency immittance for neonates: A normative study. *Acta Otolaryngologica, 127,* 49–56.

Thornton, A. R. D., Kimm, L., Kennedy, C. R., & Cafarelli-Dees, D. (1993). External- and middle-ear factors affecting evoked otoacoustic emissions in neonates. *British Journal of Audiology, 27,* 319–327.

Vanhuyse, V. J., Creten, W. L., & Van Camp, K. J. (1975). On the W-notching of tympanogram. *Scandinavian Audiology, 4,* 45–50.

Vincent, V. L., & Gerber, S. E. (1987). Early development of the acoustic reflex. *Audiology, 26,* 356–362.

Wada, H., Kobayashi, T., Suetake, M., & Tachiki, H. (1989). Dynamic behaviour of the middle ear based on sweep frequency tympanometry. *Audiology, 28*, 127–134.

Weatherby, L. A., & Bennett, M. J. (1980). The neonatal acoustic reflex. *Scandinavian Audiology, 9*, 103–110.

Williams, M. J., Purdy, S. C., & Barber, C. S. (1995). High-frequency probe tone tympanometry in infants with middle ear effusion. *Australian Journal of Otolaryngology, 2*, 169–173.

Wright, P. F., McConnell, K. B., Thompson, J. M., Vaughn, W. K., & Sell, S. H. (1985). A longitudinal study of the detection of otitis media in the first two years of life. *International Journal of Pediatric Otorhinolaryngology, 10*, 245–252.

CHAPTER 3

High-Frequency (1000 Hz) Tympanometry: Clinical Applications

JOSEPH KEI AND RAFIDAH MAZLAN

INTRODUCTION

This chapter introduces the principles and applications of high-frequency (1000 Hz) tympanometry (HFT) for evaluating the middle ear function of young infants (≤6 months). Although the use of HFT was suggested in the 1980s, its routine use with young infants in clinics did not start until the equipment became commercially available in 2000. The Joint Committee on Infant Hearing (JCIH, 2007) recommended the use of HFT in a test battery approach to assess the middle ear function of young infants, including newborns. Despite its popular use in clinics around the world, HFT does not have a universally accepted protocol. To date, no universal agreement on the interpretation of HFT findings has been made.

The chapter begins with a brief description of the principles of conventional tympanometry and HFT, followed by an outline of the commonly used test protocols and interpretation of HFT findings. The chapter concludes with case reports illustrating the application of HFT to young infants.

PRINCIPLES OF TYMPANOMETRY

Tympanometry is a measure of acoustic admittance of the middle ear as a function of air pressure change in the external ear canal (ANSI, 1987). In conventional tympanometry, it consists of the presentation of a 226-Hz tone at 85 dB SPL while the air pressure in the ear canal is changed from +200 to −400 daPa. When the probe tone is delivered into the ear canal, part of the energy is bounced back from the tympanic membrane while the rest is transmitted into the middle ear system, assuming negligibly absorption of energy by the ear canal wall. Hence, the sound pressure level inside the ear canal would decrease if no additional energy is supplied to the system. The sound pressure level inside the ear canal is measured by a probe microphone, which is connected to an electrical circuit. The electric circuit monitors the sound pressure level by supplying a voltage to adjust the output of the earphone to keep the sound pressure level constant at 85 dB SPL. The supplied voltage is directly proportional to the acoustic admittance of the middle ear system. In other words, the larger the supplied voltage, the greater is the energy flowing into the middle ear system. With appropriate calibration of the probe under standard conditions (atmospheric pressure of 1.013×10^5 Pa at 25°C at sea level), the acoustic admittance can be accurately measured in mmho. As the applied air pressure to ear canal varies from 200 to −400 daPa, the acoustic admittance is measured and plotted on a graph. The resulting graph is called a tympanogram which shows a variation of acoustic admittance, Y, against ear canal pressure.

Figure 3–1 shows a tympanogram obtained from an adult ear with normal middle ear function. Y varies depending on the ear canal pressure. Each value of Y on the tympanogram represents the sum of the admittances from the middle ear and the ear canal. Y attains a maximum value at 0 daPa, at which maximum transfer of sound energy from the ear canal to the middle ear is assumed to occur.

Although the magnitude of the acoustic admittance, Y, is shown on the tympanogram, the acoustic admittance in fact is a vector quantity having both magnitude and direction, and is represented by a bold symbol (**Y**). **Y** is made up of two components: acoustic conductance (**G**) and acoustic susceptance (**B**), which are vector quantities. [*Note:* Bolded symbols represent physical quantities with both magnitude and direction, whereas unbolded symbols refer to physical quantities with magnitude only.] The acoustic susceptance, **B**, is the difference between the stiffness (compliant) susceptance (**B$_C$**) and the mass susceptance (**B$_M$**) because **B$_C$** and **B$_M$** act against each other. The graphical representation of **Y**, **G**, and **B** is illustrated in Figure 3–2. Mathematically,

$$\boldsymbol{Y} = \boldsymbol{G} + j\boldsymbol{B} \qquad \text{Eqn. (1)}$$

where $\boldsymbol{B} = \boldsymbol{B_C} - \boldsymbol{B_M}$ and j**B** represents the vertical component which is 90° out of phase with the horizontal component **G**.

The conductance, G, is independent of the frequency (f) of sound (the probe tone). However, B_M decreases and B_C increases with increasing f as shown below.

$$B_M = 1/(2\pi f M) \qquad \text{Eqn. (2)}$$

where M is the mass of the middle ear system, and

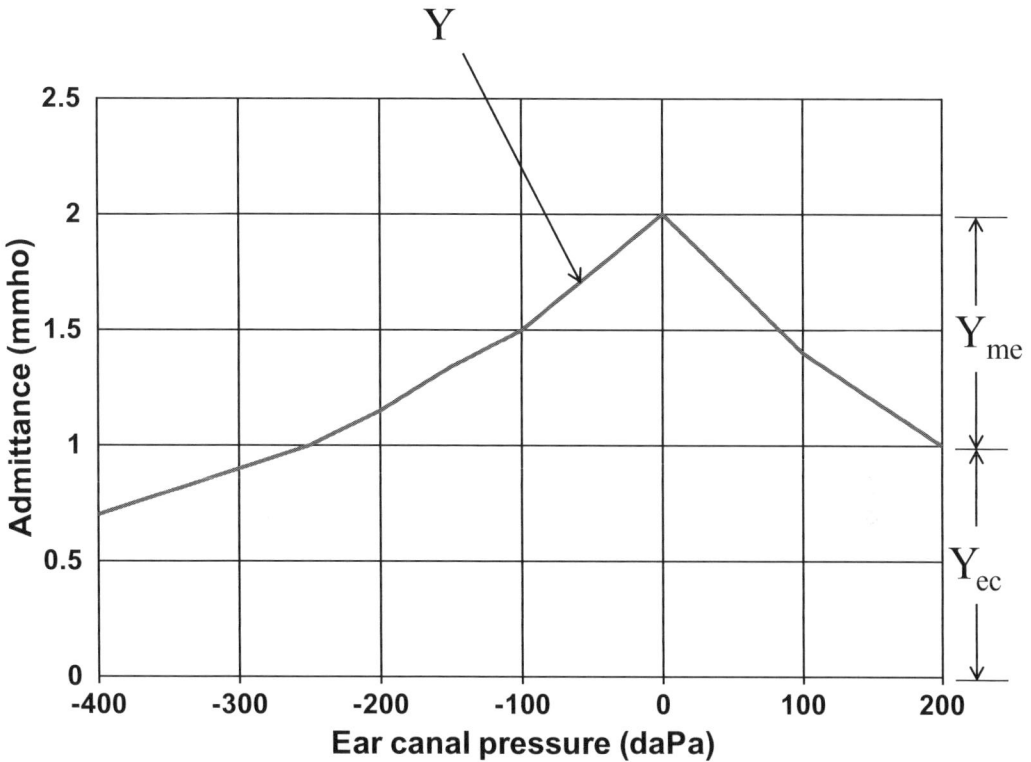

FIGURE 3–1. A tympanogram with acoustic admittance (Y) plotted against ear canal pressure obtained from an adult with normal middle ear function. Each value of Y on the tympanogram represents the sum of the admittances from the middle ear and the ear canal. At the tympanometric peak pressure (0 daPa), Y attains a maximum value of 2 mmho with contributions from the middle ear (Y_{me}) of 1 mmho and the ear canal (Y_{ec}) of 1 mmho.

$$B_C = 2\pi f V/(\rho c^2) \qquad \text{Eqn. (3)}$$

where ρ = density of air at 25°C = 1.184 kgm^{-3}, c = velocity of sound = 346.65 ms^{-1}, and V = equivalent volume of an enclosed quantity of air.

Substituting f = 226 Hz and the numerical values of ρ and c into Equation (3), the equation is reduced to:

$$B_C = 0.001V \qquad \text{Eqn. (4)}$$

If the volume is measured in cm^3 or mL, this equation can be written as:

$$B_C = V \qquad \text{Eqn. (5)}$$

That is, using a probe tone of 226 Hz, the compliance susceptance (B_C) of an enclosed volume of air is numerically equal to the volume (measured in cm^3 or mL).

Measuring Acoustic Admittance in Volume Terms

In measuring the middle ear function of a healthy ear, the acoustic admittance attains a peak value at an ear canal pressure of around 0 daPa. This peak acoustic admittance, usually called

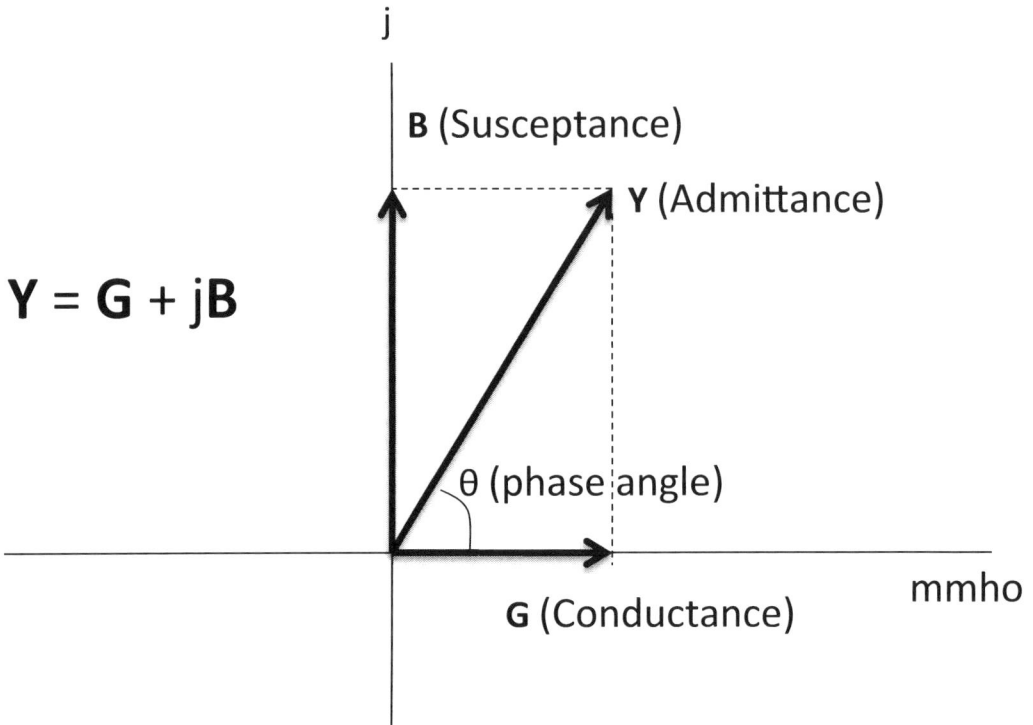

FIGURE 3–2. Acoustic admittance components, susceptance (**B**) and conductance (**G**), represented in a Cartesian coordinate system. The acoustic admittance **Y** is the sum of the susceptance and conductance components. The phase angle θ is the angle between **Y** and the horizontal axis. Mathematically, **Y** = **G** + j**B**.

"uncompensated peak acoustic admittance (Y_a)," is the sum of the admittance of the ear canal (Y_{ec}) and the admittance of the middle ear (Y_{me}) (or Y_{BC200} as abbreviated in Chapter 2).

To determine Y_{me} (also called "peak compensated static admittance"), which is an estimate of the mobility of the tympanic membrane and the middle ear system, the admittance of the ear canal has to be subtracted from the uncompensated peak admittance as shown by the following equation:

$$Y_{me} = Y_a - Y_{ec} \qquad \text{Eqn. (6)}$$

As the acoustic admittances Y_{me}, Y_a, and Y_{ec} are vector quantities, Y_{me} can only be determined accurately if both the magnitude and direction (phase angle) of Y_a and Y_{ec} are considered in the calculation. Alternatively, the mathematics can be simplified if both Y_a and Y_{ec} have the same direction (phase angle). To this end, two assumptions are made.

Assumption 1: Y_a is practically that of pure susceptance.

Assumption 2: Y_{ec} is practically that of pure susceptance.

The above two assumptions ensure that Y_a and Y_{ec} have the same phase angle. Equation (6), therefore, can be represented as:

$$Y_{me} = Y_a - Y_{ec} \qquad \text{Eqn. (7)}$$

where Y_a and Y_{ec} are scalar quantities (having magnitude only).

As $\mathbf{Y} = \mathbf{G} + j(\mathbf{B_C} - \mathbf{B_M})$ (Equation 1), Assumption 1 implies that the conductance (G) and the mass susceptance (B_M) must be very much smaller than the compliance susceptance (B_C). Mathematically, $B_C \gg G$, and $B_C \gg B_M$. Hence, Equation (1) becomes:

$$Y_a \approx B_C \qquad \text{Eqn. (8)}$$

As $B_C = V$ [Equation (5)], the acoustic admittance is numerically equal to the volume of air enclosed by the probe tip and the middle ear (V). That is,

$$Y_a \approx V \qquad \text{Eqn. (9)}$$

Hence, the acoustic admittance Y_a can be measured in volume units such as cm^3 or mL (a scalar quantity) and is commonly known as "maximum compliance." Likewise, Assumption 2 implies that Y_{ec} can also be measured in volume terms and is commonly known as "ear canal volume (V_{ec})."

In performing tympanometry on a healthy ear, Y_a will attain maximum compliance (C_{max}) at an ear canal pressure (known as tympanometric peak pressure). The static compliance (SC), which is measure of the mobility of the tympanic membrane or middle ear sys-

tem, can be deduced. Equation (7) can be transformed into:

$$SC = C_{max} - V_{ec} \qquad \text{Eqn. (10)}$$

Figure 3–3 illustrates how SC is determined from two scalar quantities, C_{max} and V_{ec}. To determine the compliance of the middle ear, it is necessary to estimate the ear canal volume. One of the methods for estimating the V_{ec} is to increase the ear canal pressure to 200 daPa and measure its equivalent volume. It is assumed that the applied pressure places the eardrum under sufficient tension as to drive the impedance of the middle ear to infinity (Assumption 3) (Terkildsen & Thompsen, 1959). That is, no sound energy can be transmitted through the tympanic membrane to the middle ear. Under this high pressure, the compliance (admittance measure at the probe tip) may be attributed to the ear canal alone, thus providing a good estimate of V_{ec}. However, several studies have demonstrated that measuring the volume at 200 daPa does not provide a good estimate of the V_{ec} (Margolis & Smith, 1977; Rabinowitz, 1981; Shanks, 1984; Shanks & Lily, 1981; Vanpeperstraete, Creten, & Van Camp, 1979). Because of the asymmetry of tympanogram, the V_{ec} measured at 200 daPa is larger than that measured at −400 daPa. Hence, the peak compensated static compliance (SC), compensated at the negative tail of −400 daPa, is larger than that compensated at the positive tail of 200 daPa (Margolis, Bass-Ringdahl, Hanks, Holte, & Zapala, 2003). Shanks and Lily (1981), as well as other researchers, proposed that measuring V_{ec}

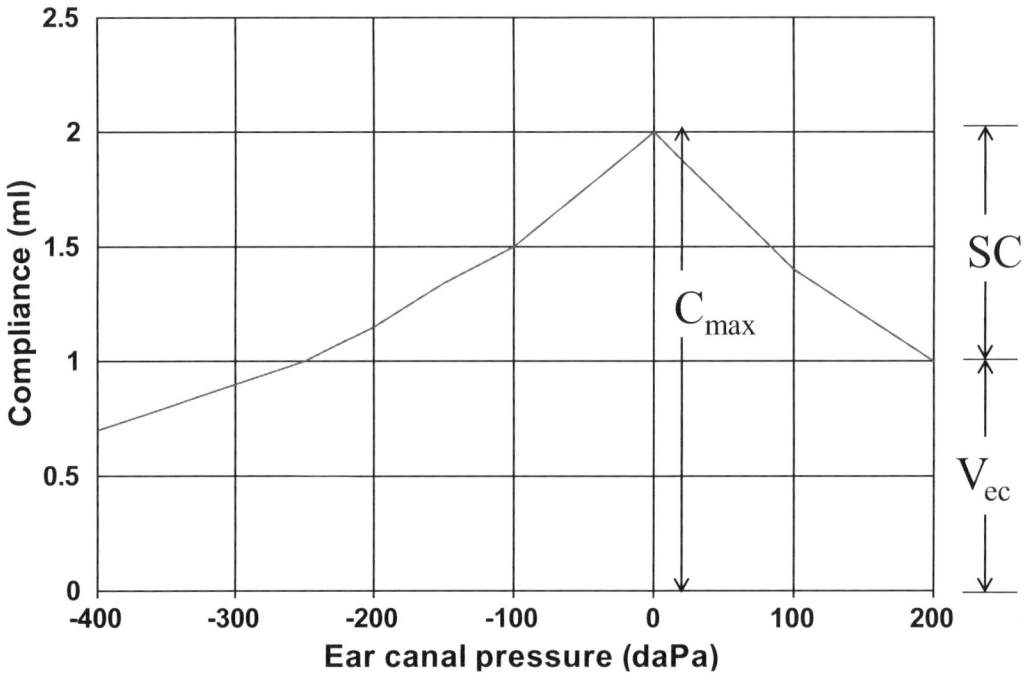

FIGURE 3–3. A tympanogram with compliance plotted against ear canal pressure obtained from an adult with normal middle ear function. At the tympanometric peak pressure (0 daPa), the compliance attains a maximum value (C_{max}) of 2 mL, which is made up of a static compliance (SC) of 1 mL and ear canal volume (V_{ec}) of 1 mL.

at –400 daPa would provide a better estimate of the volume of the ear canal than that measured at 200 daPa. Although compensation at the negative tail provides more accurate estimates of V_{ec} and, hence, a larger value of SC, it has not been widely adopted by clinicians. In fact, estimating ear canal volume at 200 daPa has been widely promoted since 1959, and has become the norm. On practical grounds, it is not always possible to estimate volume at –400 daPa because of the possibility of a collapsed ear canal. To date, there has not been enough evidence to justify that the use of compensation at the negative tail is clinically more useful than that compensated at the positive pressure end.

Application of Conventional Tympanometry

Conventional tympanometry is a useful clinical tool for identifying various disorders of the middle ear for children and adults. The sensitivity and specificity of conventional tympanometry in detecting middle ear effusion (MEE) in adults and children have been reported to be 82 to 89% and 95 to 100%, respectively (Bluestone, Beery, & Paradise, 1973; Cantekin, Bluestone, Fria, Stool, Beery, & Sabo, 1980). However, its application to neonates and young infants is questionable and is not recommended (see Chapter 2 for a brief review).

HIGH-FREQUENCY (1000) TYMPANOMETRY (HFT)

The use of HFT with a probe tone of 1 kHz did not start until 2000 when the equipment became commercially available. Since then, clinicians have begun to explore the characteristics of HFT and establish normative data for neonates and young infants. Although normative HFT data are emerging, there have been discrepancies in the HFT measurements to date. Most importantly, the way to analyze and interpret HFT findings in neonates has not universally been agreed upon. Presently, the calibration of the HFT equipment is based on measurements of acoustic admittance magnitude and phase angle using a 226-Hz tone in a 2-mL calibration cavity. It is not clear if it is more appropriate to calibrate HFT instruments using a probe tone of 1 kHz instead. The following sections outline the development of the HFT, including the principles, procedures, and methods of interpreting HFT data.

Principles of High-Frequency Tympanometry

Theoretically, the principles of HFT do not appear to be different from those of conventional tympanometry. Equations (1) and (6) apply equally well to both conventional tympanometry and HFT. Previous investigations using high frequency tympanometric techniques (e.g., using probe tones of 678 Hz and 1 kHz) mainly focused on conductance (G) and susceptance (B) measurements and their

interpretation of results using the Vanhuyse model (Vanhuyse, Creten, & Van Camp, 1975). Although this model was valuable in classifying multipeaked tympanometric patterns, it did not provide adequate clinical information. Kei et al. (2003) and Margolis et al. (2003) were the first to analyze HFT results based on acoustic admittance measures. In particular, Kei et al. (2003) found that 92.2% of 122 newborn babies in the well nursery ward exhibited clear single-peaked admittance patterns, with another 5.7% showing a shallow single-peaked admittance tympanogram. Multiple-peaked admittance tympanograms were rare in newborn babies when a probe tone of 1 kHz was used. The implication of these findings is that HFT results can be classified in a way similar to that of the Jerger (1970) classification for conventional tympanometry.

METHODS FOR INTERPRETING HFT RESULTS

Three methods are currently used to interpret HFT findings. These methods include: (1) examination of the morphology only; (2) morphology plus baseline compensated static admittance; and (3) morphology plus component compensated static admittance.

Examination of the Morphology Method

Baldwin (2006) examined the morphology (shape) of acoustic admittance tympanograms to categorize HFT results. In her study of HFT on 211 babies aged 2 to 21 weeks, tympanograms recorded from babies with normal ABR thresholds or robust transient evoked otoacoustic emissions (TEOAEs) were compared with those recorded from infants who had evidence of conductive hearing impairment attributed to middle ear effusion (MEE). Using a shape classification method adapted from Marchant, McMillan, Shurin, Johnson, Turczyk, Feinstein, and Panek (1986), the tympanograms were analyzed by drawing a line between the admittance values at +300 daPa and −400 daPa and examining the shape of tympanograms referenced to the line. Baldwin (2006) then classified tympanograms into two major categories: results with a positive peak from the line were considered normal; and those with a negative peak (or trough) configuration were classified as abnormal. In classifying HFT tympanograms, Baldwin (2006) found that 5% of traces were difficult to classify in the "normal" group and 0.6% in the "MEE" group. In view of this difficulty, clinicians should exercise care in interpreting HFT results for these borderline cases. Moreover, the diagnosis should be made in conjunction with other tests such as otoacoustic emission and acoustic stapedial reflex tests.

Using this morphology only method, Baldwin (2006) established the sensitivity and specificity of the HFT for correctly identifying the presence of MEE to be 0.99 and 0.89, respectively. In another study, Swanepoel, Werner, Hugo, Louw, Owen, and Swanepoel (2007) compared distortion product otoacoustic emission test outcomes (pass/refer) with HFT outcomes (peak/no peak) obtained from 278 neonates aged from 0 to 4 weeks. Acknowledging that OAEs are not a perfect gold standard for comparison, they found that the sensitivity and specificity of the HFT for detecting middle ear pathology were 57% and 95%, respectively.

Morphology Plus Baseline Compensated Static Admittance Method

This method, advocated by Kei et al. (2003) and Margolis et al. (2003), examines both the morphology of the traces and peak compensated static admittance. Most HFT devices (e.g., the Madsen Capella, Madsen Otoflex 100, Grason-Stadler GSI-33, and GSI Tymstar tympanometers) display a tympanogram similar to that shown in Figure 3–4, which shows a tympanogram obtained from a 2-day-old baby boy with robust otoacoustic emissions. The static admittance, compensated for the ear canal effect at an ear canal pressure of 200 daPa, was 0.75 mmho which is within the 90% range (0.23 to 1.35 mmho) reported by Mazlan, Kei, Hickson, Gavranich, and Linning (2009b). In addition to examining the morphology of the tympanogram, this method provides an objective measure of the peak compensated static admittance. This measure is important to distinguish normal from abnormal HFT results, especially when a tympanogram with a small positive peak is obtained.

Alternatively, the acoustic admittance can be compensated for ear canal effect from the negative tail (−400 daPa). Based on data from 30 full-term babies aged from 2 to 4 weeks, Margolis and

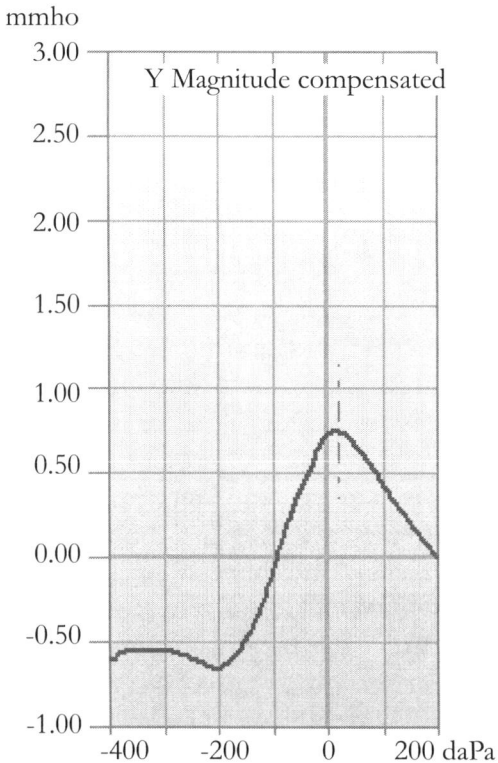

FIGURE 3–4. A tympanogram obtained from a 2-day-old male. The results show good morphology (a single positive peak) with peak compensated static admittance (compensated for the ear canal effect at +200 daPa) of 0.75 mmho.

colleagues (2003) established a pass criterion of static admittance compensated at the negative tail of at least 0.6 mmho (5th percentile) using the Grason-Stadler GSI-33 (Version 2) device. Although the static admittance compensated at the negative tail of −400 daPa is usually larger than that compensated at the positive tail of 200 daPa, the accuracy of this measure may be affected by the presence of a collapsed ear canal before the ear canal pressure reaches −400 daPa (Kei, Mazlan, Hickson, Gavranich, & Linning, 2007).

Regardless of where the compensation takes place, the above method of interpreting tympanograms offers an additional dimension in assessing the middle ear status of young infants. However, in estimating the static admittance of the middle ear, errors may be involved, as shown by Equation (6): $Y_{me} = Y_a - Y_{ec}$. In the calculation, the uncompensated peak admittance (Y_a) and admittance at either the positive or the negative end (Y_{ec}) are assumed to have the same phase angle [$\theta = \tan^{-1} (B/G)$]. That is, both Y_a and Y_{ec} are stiffness dominated and pointing in the same upward direction (i.e., the phase angles of Y_a and Y_{ec} are close to 90°). Although this is true when adults and older children are tested using 226-Hz tympanometry, this is not the case when 1000 Hz tympanometry is applied to young infants. In reality, when the HFT is applied to young infants who have a mass dominated middle ear system, Y_a and Y_{ec} are pointing in a more horizontal direction and the directions are different (Kei et al., 2007). According to Kei and colleagues (2007), this magnitude compensated static admittance method yields a smaller Y_{me} (Y_{BC200}) value than that derived from a component compensated static admittance method which takes both the magnitude and direction of Y_a and Y_{ec} into consideration.

Morphology Plus Component Compensated Static Admittance Method

This method, advocated by Alaerts, Luts, and Wouters (2007), Calandruccio, Fitzgerald, and Prieve (2006), Kei et al.

(2007), and Mazlan et al. (2009b), examines both the morphology of the traces and component compensated static admittance. Although the way to examine the morphology remains unchanged (positive peak versus no peak or trough), the approach to measure the peak compensated static admittance (of the middle ear) is different. As mentioned above, errors may be involved in deriving Y_{me} if Y_a and Y_{ec} are not compensated for both magnitude and direction (Kei et al., 2007; Margolis & Hunter, 2000). As recommended by Margolis and Hunter (2000) and Kei et al. (2007), it is necessary to calculate compensated conductance and susceptance separately when a 1000-Hz probe tone is used. The compensated conductance G_{me} and susceptance B_{me} are:

$$G_{me} = G_{peak} - G_{tail} \qquad \text{Eqn. (11)}$$

$$B_{me} = B_{peak} - B_{tail} \qquad \text{Eqn. (12)}$$

where B_{tail} and G_{tail} represent the susceptance and conductance at +200 daPa, respectively; and B_{peak} and G_{peak} represent uncompensated peak susceptance and conductance, respectively. From the compensated conductance and susceptance, the component compensated static admittance, which is denoted as Y_{mecc} [or Y_{CC200} as abbreviated in Chapter 2], can be determined using the following equation:

$$Y_{mecc} = \sqrt{(G_{me}{}^2 + B_{me}{}^2)} \qquad \text{Eqn. (13)}$$

In this approach, the admittance at +200 daPa (Y_{ec}) is calculated using the equation:

$$Y_{ec} = \sqrt{(G_{tail}{}^2 + B_{tail}{}^2)} \qquad \text{Eqn. (14)}$$

The graphic representation of this method (the component compensated admittance approach) is available from the Madsen Otoflex 100 device as shown in Figure 3–5. The tympanogram showing the component compensated static admittance plotted against ear canal pressure is different from that of the magnitude (baseline) compensated admittance approach. Although the magnitude compensated admittance attains a negative admittance value when the ear canal pressure decreases to below −100 daPa, the component compensated admittance assumes a positive value regardless of the ear canal pressure. Kei et al. (2007) and Mazlan et al. (2009b) found that the mean component compensated static admittance (Y_{mecc}) (or Y_{CC200}) was always greater than the mean magnitude compensated static admittance (Y_{me}) (or Y_{BC200}). They concluded that the larger mean admittance values of the component compensated static admittance may allow a better separation of abnormal tympanograms from the normal ones.

Presently, the above three methods have been utilized by clinicians around the world. It is not clear if one particular method is better than the others in diagnosing MEE in young infants. More research investigating the test performance of HFT using various methods needs to be determined in future studies.

NORMATIVE HFT DATA

Given the widespread implementation of universal newborn hearing screening programs and the ability of HFT to

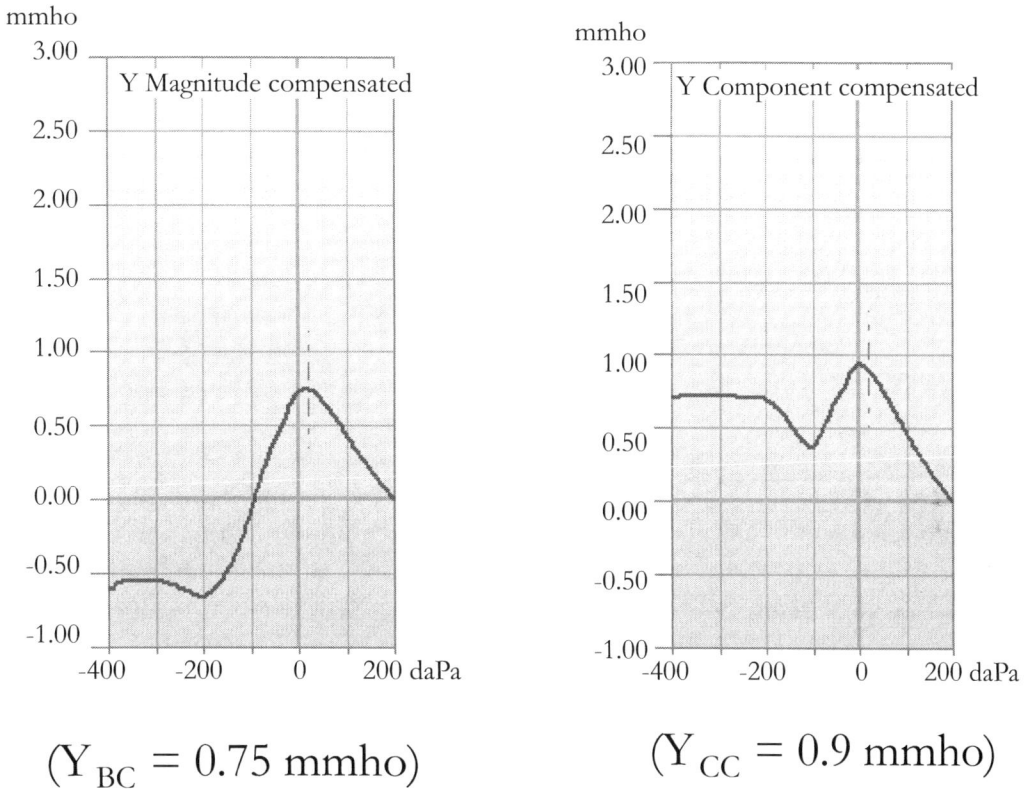

$$(Y_{BC} = 0.75 \text{ mmho})$$

$$(Y_{CC} = 0.9 \text{ mmho})$$

FIGURE 3–5. Tympanograms obtained from the same neonate using two different methods. The diagram on the left shows a tympanogram obtained using the conventional magnitude (baseline) compensated admittance method. The right tympanogram was obtained using the component compensated admittance method. Although the magnitude compensated admittance attains a negative admittance value when the ear canal pressure decreases to below –100 daPa, the component compensated admittance assumes a positive value regardless of the ear canal pressure. The peak compensated static admittances for the magnitude and component compensated methods were 0.75 and 0.90 mmho, respectively.

detect middle ear dysfunction in neonates (Margolis et al., 2003; Purdy & Williams, 2000; Rhodes, Margolis, Hirsch, & Napp, 1999; Williams, Purdy, & Barber, 1995), there is a pressing need to establish normative data using both the magnitude (baseline) and component compensation approaches. Presently, there is no guideline on which HFT parameters should be included in collecting normative data. Recent normative studies show a propensity for the peak compensated static admittance (including either the magnitude or component compensation) to be used as the main test parameter in examining HFT data. Other test parameters such as the tympanometric peak pressure (TPP), uncompensated peak admittance (Y) and admittance at +200 daPa (Y_{200}) have been reported in most normative studies (Alaerts et al., 2007; Calandruccio et al., 2006; Kei et al., 2003; Kei et al., 2007; Margolis et al., 2003; Mazlan et al.,

2007; Mazlan et al., 2009b; Swanepoel et al., 2007). At this stage, it is not clear how important these other parameters are in the interpretation of HFT results. Nevertheless, the normative data showing the 90% range of these parameters, described in Table 3–1, may serve as a reference to assist in the interpretation of HFT results.

Table 3–1 shows a summary of findings of the normative studies published during the 2003 to 2009 period. For comparison purposes, the HFT results obtained by Kei et al. (2003) were collapsed across the left and right ears. As shown in Table 3–1, the TPP values are quite variable with mean TPP obtained by Mazlan et al. (2009b) being significantly greater than that obtained by either Margolis et al. (2003) or Swanepoel et al. (2007). The Y_{200} values also vary from study to study, with mean Y_{200} obtained from the Mazlan et al. (2009b) study being significantly smaller than that from either the Margolis et al. (2003) or Kei et al. (2003) study. The mean uncompensated peak admittance, Y, obtained by Mazlan et al. (2009b) was significantly smaller than that obtained by either Margolis et al. (2003) or Swanepoel et al. (2007). The mean magnitude compensated static admittance, Y_{me}, obtained by Mazlan et al. (2009b) was significantly smaller than that obtained by Margolis et al. (2003), but greater than that obtained by Kei et al. (2003). The comparison of Y_{mecc} obtained by Mazlan et al. (2009b) with that by Alaerts et al. (2007) or Calandruccio et al. (2006) is not possible as the mean and standard deviation values are not available. Nevertheless,

the median and 90% ranges reported by the three studies appear to be similar.

There is general consensus that age is significant factor in HFT findings with Y, Y_{200}, Y_{me}, and Y_{mecc} increasing with age, especially during the first six months of life (e.g., Alaerts et al., 2007; Calandruccio et al., 2006; Mazlan et al., 2007; Swanepoel et al., 2007). No gender or ear differences are found, apart from a possible ear asymmetry effect reported by Kei et al. (2003).

Overall, there are significant differences in the HFT normative data between studies. A number of factors could have contributed to these differences. First, there are differences in instrumentation. Devices with different probe design can affect HFT results. For example, the probe and tips used in the Madsen Capella were found to be too large for newborn babies. The Y_{200} values obtained from newborn babies using this device were greater than those obtained using the Madsen Otoflex 100 (Mazlan et al., 2007). The Madsen Otoflex 100 was found to provide better probe fit for neonates than the Madsen Capella.

Second, different test protocols can have a significant impact on the HFT result and its interpretation. However, a universally accepted test protocol for HFT, to date, has not been established. For example, the protocol used by Calandruccio et al. (2006) involves delivering a 1000-Hz probe tone at 85 dB SPL to the ear with applied air pressure in the ear canal varying at a pump speed of 125 daPa/s. Margolis et al. (2003) and Swanepoel et al. (2007) used Grason-Stadler GSI-33 and Tymstar (Version 2)

TABLE 3–1. Summary of Findings of the Normative Studies Published During the 2003 to 2009 Period

Study	N (ears)	Age	Equipment	TPP (daPa)	Y_{200} (mmho)	Y (mmho)	Y_{me} (mmho)	Y_{mecc} (mmho)
Kei et al. (2003)	106	1–6 days	Madsen Capella	18.3 (41.6) [−58–87]	1.6 (0.6) [0.7–2.5]	2.1 NA [0.9–3.6]	0.6 (0.3) [0.2–1.1]	NA NA NA
Margolis et al. (2003)	46	14–28 days	Grason-Stadler GSI-33 (ver. 2)	−10.0 (68.0) [−133–113]	1.4 (0.4) [0.8–2.2]	2.7 (1.2) [0.8–4.8]	1.3 (1.0) [0.1–3.5]	NA NA NA
Calandruccio et al. (2006)	39	4–10 weeks	Virtual Model 310	NA NA	Med = 1.3 [1.0–1.7]	NA NA	NA NA	Med = 1.1 [0.2–2.3]
	39	11–19 weeks		NA NA	Med = 1.4 [1.1–1.9]	NA NA	NA NA	Med = 1.5 [0.7–2.3]
Alaerts et al. (2007)	15	< 3 months	Madsen Otoflex 100	Med = 7.0 [−96–86]	Med = 1.1 [0.6–1.8]	NA NA	NA NA	Med = 1.0 [0.3–2.7]
	30	3–9 months		Med = −52 [−126–13]	Med = 2.0 [1.4–3.1]	NA NA	NA NA	Med = 1.9 [0.8–3.6]

continues

TABLE 3–1. *continued*

Study	N (ears)	Age	Equipment	TPP (daPa)	Y_200 (mmho)	Y (mmho)	Y_me (mmho)	Y_mecc (mmho)
Swanepoel et al. (2007)	73	1–7 days	Grason-Stadler GSI-Tymstar (ver. 2)	−10.0	NA	2.2	NA	NA
				(48.0)	NA	(0.9)	NA	NA
				[−70–70]	NA	[1.2–3.4]	NA	NA
	177	1–4 weeks		5.0	NA	2.4	NA	NA
				(49.0)	NA	(0.7)	NA	NA
				[−80–85]	NA	[1.5–3.8]	NA	NA
Mazlan et al. (2009b)	157	1–8 days	Madsen Otoflex 100	13.5	1.0	1.7	0.7	1.0
				(49.4)	(0.4)	(0.7)	(0.3)	(0.5)
				Med = 13.0	Med = 1.0	Med = 1.6	Med = 0.6	Med = 0.9
				[−73–89]	[0.5–1.7]	[0.9–2.8]	[0.2–1.4]	[0.4–1.9]

Mean and SD values (in parenthesis) or median (Med), and 90% range (in square brackets) are shown.

SD = standard deviation; Med = median; NA = not available; TPP = tympanometric peak pressure; Y = uncompensated peak admittance; Y_{200} = admittance at +200 daPa; Y_{me} = magnitude compensated static admittance; Y_{mecc} = component compensated static admittance.

to deliver a 1000-Hz probe tone (presumably at 85 dB SPL, but not reported by the authors) to the ear with applied air pressure varying from 600 daPa/s at the tails to 200 daPa/s near the peak. Kei et al. (2003) and Mazlan et al. (2009b) utilized a 1000-Hz probe tone at 75 dB SPL and a higher pump speed of 400 daPa/s. In the tiny ears of newborn babies with an ear canal volume of approximately 0.2 to 0.4 mL, the difference of 10 dB in probe tone levels can have a considerable effect on the acoustical properties of the auditory system. This is particularly important for neonates who have low acoustic stapedial reflex thresholds (e.g., <80 dB HL) for the tonal stimuli (Mazlan, Kei, & Hickson, 2009a).

Third, different age groups may produce dissimilar normative data. As the auditory system develops rapidly in the first 6 months of life, the HFT normative data must be age-specific, with a narrow age range for each age group. More research to collect age-specific data is needed in future to assit clinicians in assessing the middle ear function of young infants. Special attention should be given to the inclusion criteria for selection of participants for the normative study (Margolis et al., 2003; Swanepoel et al., 2007).

Fourth, the calibration of the HFT devices can affect the accuracy of the measurements (Mazlan et al., 2009b). Currently, the calibration is based on measurements of acoustic admittance magnitude and phase angle using a 226-Hz tone in three calibration cavities with volumes of 0.5, 2, and 5 mL. In the calibration process, the admittance magnitude and phase indicators are adjusted to read 0.5, 2, and 5 mmho with a phase angle of 90 degrees for all three cavities. The requirement of the 90-degree phase angle implies that the enclosed cavity is nearly an ideal compliant element, consisting of a positive susceptance value and a conductance of 0 mmho (Margolis & Hunter, 2000). Although such calibration standard is valid for conducting 226-Hz tympanometry for adults and older children, it is not certain if it is appropriate for calibrating HFT devices that utilize a probe tone of 1000 Hz for all measurements. It would be of prime clinical importance to compare middle ear admittance values obtained using different instruments on the same cohort of newborn babies in future studies to check if HFT normative data are instrument-specific or not. Given the prime importance of calibration on HFT measurements, it is imperative to have a unified calibration standard and test protocol for assessing middle ear function in young infants.

Finally, the normative HFT data may depend on the demographic characteristics (e.g., race and age) of participants. Normative HFT data should be collected for different races and some special populations such as indigenous children who have a high prevalence of otitis media (Boswell & Nienhuys, 1995).

Although normative HFT data can inform clinicians of the range of normal values of some important test parameters, they are based on the statistical analysis of data collected from infants with normal auditory function and, therefore, do not provide comprehensive diagnostic information on middle ear pathology. Further research to investigate the relationship between the type of middle ear disorders and pattern of HFT results is warranted. Determination of the test performance of HFT in identifying middle ear pathology in a large sample of age-specific young infants is imperative.

Suggested Protocol for Performing HFT in Young Infants

There is clear evidence that HFT with a probe tone of 1000 Hz should be used with young infants (Alaerts et al., 2007; Calandruccio et al., 2006). Older infants (> 6 months) would require conventional tympanometry with a probe tone of 226 Hz. Unlike conventional tympanometry, which is used with older children and adults, the intensity level of the probe tone in HFT should be less than 85 dB SPL. In the ear of a neonate with ear canal volume of 0.2 to 0.4 ml, a 1000-Hz probe tone of 85 dB SPL (81.5 dB HL as measured in a 2-mL cavity) would be high enough to elicit an acoustic stapedial reflex, especially when the neonate has low reflex thresholds. The stapedial reflex alters the impedance of the middle ear and, hence, the shape of the tympanogram. To reduce this possibility, a probe tone of 75 dB SPL (71.5 dB HL) is recommended. Additionally, the applied ear canal pressure should vary from a positive pressure of +200 daPa to a negative pressure of −400 daPa (or even −300 daPa to cause less discomfort to young infants). It is not necessary to extend the pressure range to −600 daPa because

a neonate's ear canal wall is so flaccid that it would have collapsed even before reaching −400 daPa. A pump speed of 300 to 400 daPa/s for the applied air pressure is appropriate to enable the test to be completed in the shortest possible time, while maintaining accuracy in recording the tympanogram.

When a single-peaked admittance tympanogram is obtained from a young infant, normal middle ear function is assumed. However, when the tympanometric peak appears too low or too high when compared to normative data, indicating possible abnormal results, the test should be repeated to check for test-retest reliability. If the same pattern of result is obtained in the repeated trial, the value of the peak compensated static admittance (magnitude or component compensated) should be checked against relevant normative data (preferably collected from the same equipment) before making a diagnosis. In any case, the diagnosis of middle ear dysfunction should be made in conjunction with other tests such as the OAEs, ABR (air and bone conduction) and acoustic stapedial reflex test.

CASE STUDIES ILLUSTRATING DIFFERENT PATTERNS OF HFT RESULTS

The cases reported in this section are babies assessed between 2009 and 2010. The purpose for showing these cases is to delineate different patterns of magnitude compensated and component compensated admittance tympanograms, obtained from neonates with and without middle ear dysfunction. In the case studies described below, only one ear was tested. The AABR was performed by an experienced midwife trained in the use of a screening device (Natus ALGO 3) as part of the Healthy Hearing Program conducted in Queensland, Australia. The two-tier AABR screening protocol resulted in a refer rate of 1.1% (Queensland Health, 2007). After the hearing screening, the authors tested the babies using TEOAE, HFT, and acoustic stapedial reflex (ASR) tests as part of a research project. The diagnosis of middle ear dysfunction was made in conjunction with other objective assessment tools including AABR, TEOAE, and ASR tests. These cases, mostly chosen from babies with possible middle ear dysfunction, are by no means representative sample of patients. Nevertheless, they do illustrate the application, analysis, and interpretation of HFT findings. In particular, we present a few borderline cases where HFT findings were ambiguous and not conclusive. Instrumentations for this research include an ILO 292 Otodynamics Analyser (OAE system software ILO, Version 5.6, Release Y) for the TEOAE test, and a Madsen Otoflex 100 (Type 1012) Otodiagnostic Suite immittance meter (GN Otometrics) for the HFT and ASR tests.

The pass criterion for the TEOAE test was at least 3 dB signal-to-noise (SNR) in at least four out of five half-octave bands centered at 1, 1.5, 2, 3, and 4 kHz (Mazlan et al., 2009b). The pass criterion for the HFT test was a single-peaked admittance tympanogram with either a magnitude compensated static

admittance of at least 0.2 mmho or a component compensated static admittance of at least 0.4 mmho (Mazlan et al., 2009b). A pass for the ASR test was awarded if the ipsilateral stapedial reflex threshold was less than 95 dB HL for the 2-kHz tone and less than 85 dB HL for the broadband noise (BBN) stimulus (Mazlan et al., 2009a).

Case 1

The baby, KH, was a female with gestational age 38.5 weeks and birth weight 3.84 kg. The birth was uneventful. She passed the newborn hearing screening conducted by Queensland Health. With her parents' written consent, she participated in a research project that investigated middle ear function. As only one ear was tested, the most accessible ear (the right ear) was selected. She was tested at 2 days of age. She slept during the test with very little jaw movement. She had robust TEOAEs (SNRs were 7, 21, 22, 21, and 19 dB at 1, 1.5, 2, 3, and 4 kHz, respectively). Ipsilateral acoustic stapedial reflex thresholds for the 2 kHz and BBN stimuli were 80 and 55 dB HL, respectively. Her HFT results, shown in Figure 3–6, indicate normal findings. The magnitude compensated tympanogram showed a single peak with middle ear admittance of 0.83 mmho at a TPP of 77 daPa. The component compensated tympanogram showed a single peak at the same TPP with middle ear admittance of 1.40 mmho. These patterns of HFT results are typical of ears with normal middle ear function during the neonatal period.

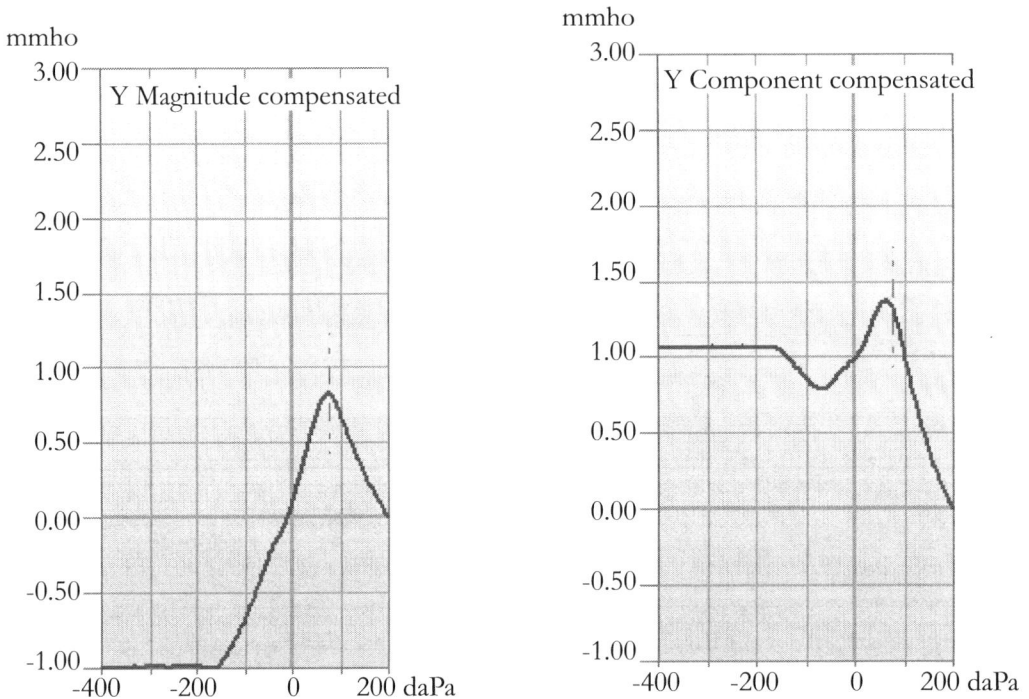

FIGURE 3–6. Tympanograms obtained from the right ear of a 2-day-old female (KH), who passed the AABR, TEOAE, and ASR tests. The results showed good morphology with normal peak compensated static admittance using either the magnitude or component compensated method.

Case 2

The baby, JB, was a male with gestational age 39 weeks and birth weight 3.3 kg. The birth was uneventful. He passed the newborn hearing screening conducted by Queensland Health. He was 2 days old at time of assessment and was asleep during the test. TEOAEs were absent (SNR ≤ 0 dB) in the left ear. Ipsilateral acoustic stapedial reflexes were absent. His HFT results, shown in Figure 3–7, indicate abnormal findings. The magnitude compensated tympanogram showed no identifiable peak with a shallow curve sloping to nega-

tive admittance values as the pressure decreased. The component compensated tympanogram showed a shallow rising curve with no identifiable peak. These patterns of HFT results are typical of ears with middle ear dysfunction during the neonatal period.

Case 3

The baby, IR, was a male with gestational age 39.6 weeks and birth weight 3.7 kg. The birth was uneventful. He passed the newborn hearing screening conducted by Queensland Health. He was 2 days old at time of assess-

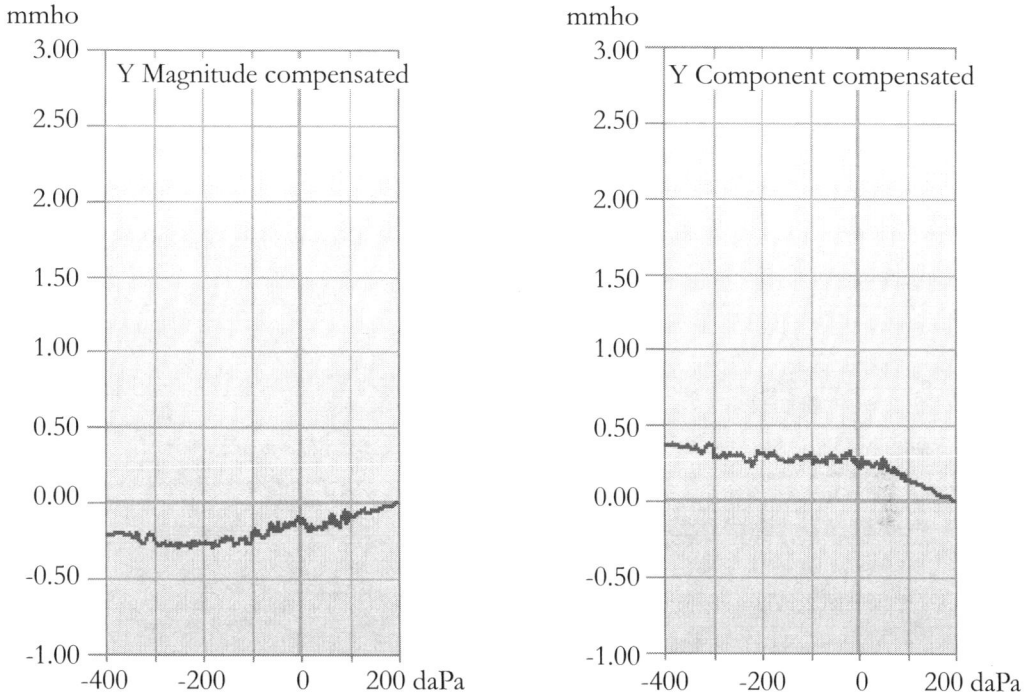

FIGURE 3–7. Tympanograms obtained from the left ear of a 2-day-old male (JB), who passed the AABR screen, but failed the TEOAE and ASR tests. The results showed poor morphology with no identifiable peak, which is a clear abnormal HFT finding.

ment and was asleep during the test. He passed the TEOAE test, but emissions were not robust (SNRs were < 0, 4, 8, 14, and 17 dB at 1, 1.5, 2, 3, and 4 kHz, respectively) in the left ear. Acoustic stapedial reflexes were absent. His HFT results, shown in Figure 3–8, indicate abnormal findings. The magnitude compensated tympanogram showed a single peak on a curve gently sloping to negative admittance values as the pressure decreased. The component compensated tympanogram showed a straight line with increasing admittance as the ear canal pressure was decreased. These patterns of HFT results, although not typical, are consistent with middle ear dysfunction. This diagnosis was

made based on the findings from the above battery of tests:

■ Passing the AABR test does not exclude the possibility of a slight to mild conductive or cochlear hearing loss;

■ Passing TEOAE with less robust emissions especially in the low to mid frequencies (1 to 2 kHz) does not exclude the possibility of conductive hearing impairment;

■ Absence of ipsilateral ASR indicates the possibility of *at least* a slight (16 to 25 dB HL) conductive hearing loss, a severe (71 to 90 dB HL) cochlear loss, or neural loss (e.g., auditory dyssynchrony) of any degree;

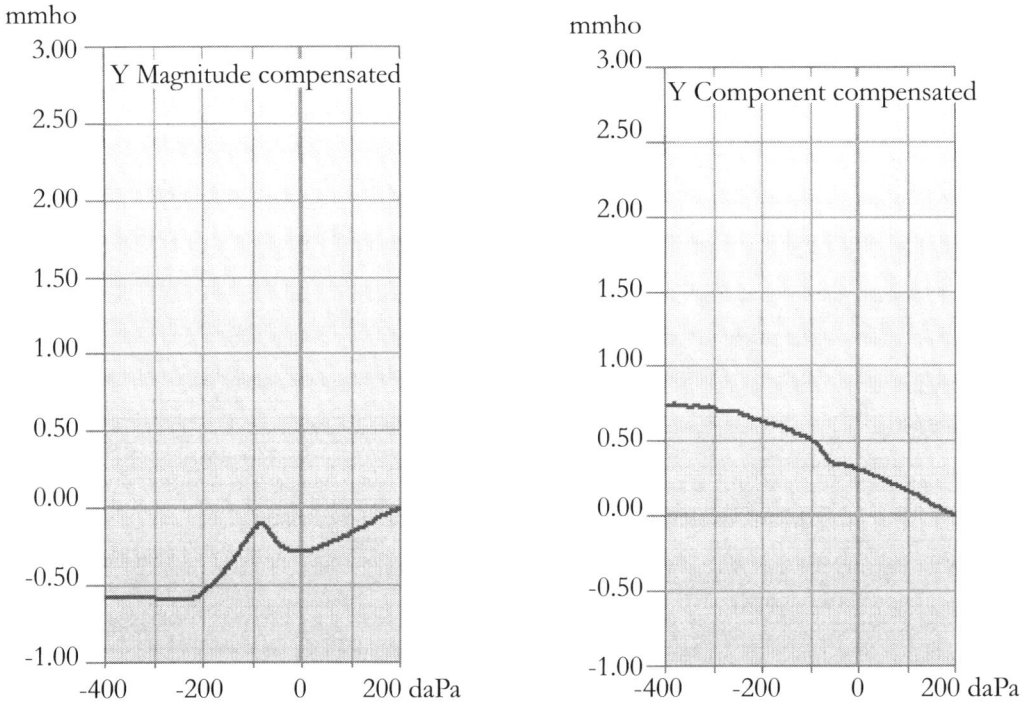

FIGURE 3–8. Tympanograms obtained from the left ear of a 2-day-old male (IR), who passed the AABR screen and the TEOAE test with less robust emissions especially in the low to mid frequencies (1–2 kHz). However, ipsilateral ASR was absent. The magnitude compensated tympanogram (*left diagram*) shows a single peak on a curve with negative admittance values. The morphology for the component compensated tympanogram is poor. Based on all the findings, IR might have a subtle middle ear problem in his left ear.

▨ Atypical HFT results indicate the possibility of middle ear dysfunction.

Combining all the above test findings, the possibility of a slight conductive hearing loss cannot be excluded.

Case 4

The baby, LJ, was a male with gestational age 38.5 weeks and birth weight 4.8 kg. The birth was uneventful. He passed the newborn hearing screening conducted by Queensland Health. He was tested while asleep at the age of 2 days. He had robust TEOAEs (SNRs were 6, 14, 18, 26, and 14 dB at 1, 1.5, 2, 3, and 4 kHz, respectively) in his left ear. Ipsilateral acoustic stapedial reflex thresholds for the 2 kHz and BBN stimuli were 60 and less than 50 dB HL, respectively. His HFT results, shown in Figure 3–9, indicate a double-peaked tympanogram. This finding, although atypical, is not conclusive in contributing to a diagnosis. In the magnitude compensated tympanogram, the higher peak was measured, showing an admittance of 0.52 mmho at a TPP of 32 daPa.

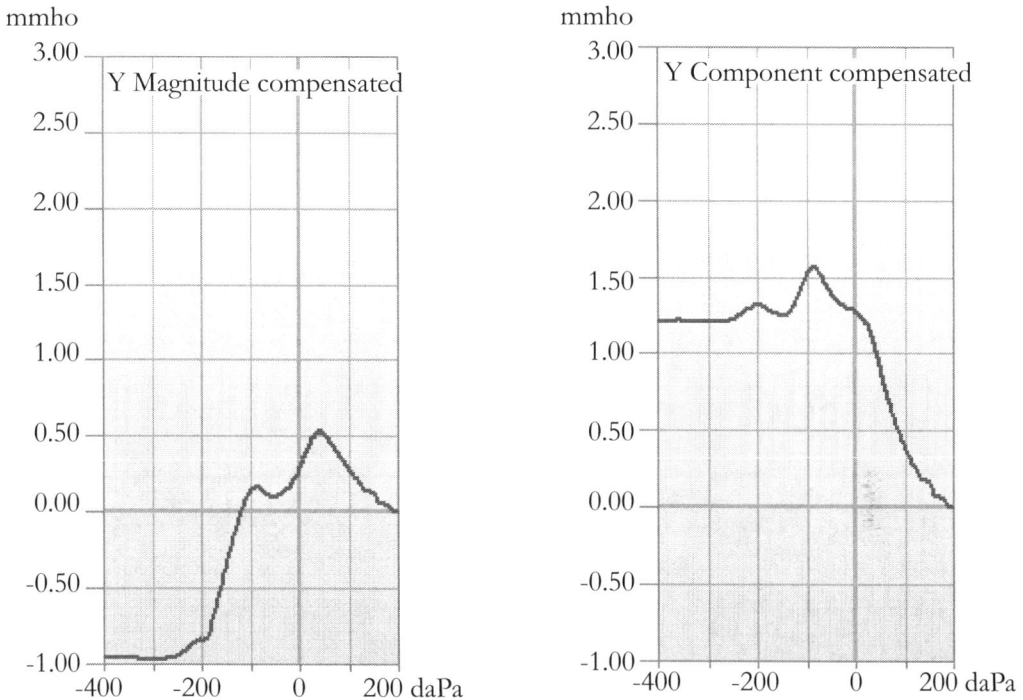

FIGURE 3–9. Tympanograms obtained from the left ear of a 2-day-old male (LJ), who passed the AABR, TEOAE, and ASR tests. The HFT results show a double-peaked pattern which is inconclusive. However, based on all the test results, LJ should have normal middle ear function.

The component compensated tympanogram showed middle ear admittance of 1.20 mmho at the same TPP. These HFT results, together with normal AABR, TEOAE, and ASR findings, are consistent with normal auditory function up to the brainstem.

Case 5

The baby, JF, was a male with gestational age 39 weeks and birth weight 3.5 kg. The birth was uneventful. He passed the newborn hearing screening conducted by Queensland Health. He was 2 days old at the time of assess-

ment and was asleep during the test. TEOAEs were absent (SNR ≤ 0 dB) in the left ear. Ipsilateral acoustic stapedial reflexes were absent. His HFT results are shown in Figure 3–10. The magnitude compensated tympanogram showed a single peak with middle ear admittance of 0.15 mmho at 40 daPa TPP. The component compensated tympanogram showed a shallow peak with middle ear admittance of 0.2 mmho at the same TPP. These HFT results, together with normal AABR findings but absent TEOAEs and absent ASRs, suggest the possibility of a subtle middle ear dysfunction.

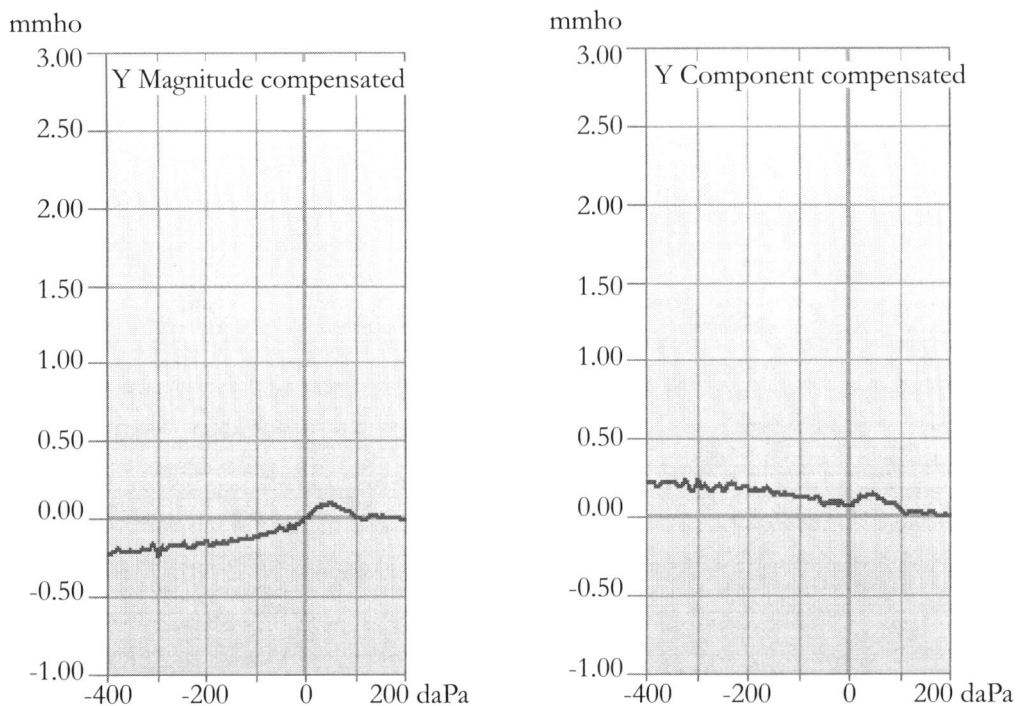

FIGURE 3–10. Tympanograms obtained from the left ear of a 2-day-old male (JF), who passed the AABR screen, but failed the TEOAE and ASR tests. Both tympanograms show a shallow positive peak, with peak compensated static admittance values falling below the 5th percentile of the normative data. Given the above results, JF may have a subtle middle ear dysfunction.

Case 6

The baby, RM, was a female with a gestational age of 41.3 weeks and birth weight of 3.7 kg. She passed the newborn hearing screening using AABR. She was tested 3 days after birth and was asleep during the test. Her left ear showed robust TEOAEs (SNRs were 11, 13, 22, 27, and 22 dB at 1, 1.5, 2, 3, and 4 kHz, respectively). Ipsilateral acoustic stapedial reflex thresholds for the 2 kHz and BBN stimuli were 60 and 50 dB HL, respectively. The magnitude compensated tympanogram, shown in Figure 3–11, showed a single peak with

middle ear admittance of 0.16 mmho at a TPP of 60 daPa. The component compensated tympanogram showed a shallow peak with middle ear admittance of 0.25 mmho at the same TPP. These HFT results, strictly speaking, would be regarded as abnormal findings according to the pass criteria. However, given that RM passed the AABR screening, and TEOAE and ASR tests, she should have normal auditory function up to the brainstem region. This special case illustrates the importance of a test battery approach to interpret HFT findings in conjunction with the findings of other tests.

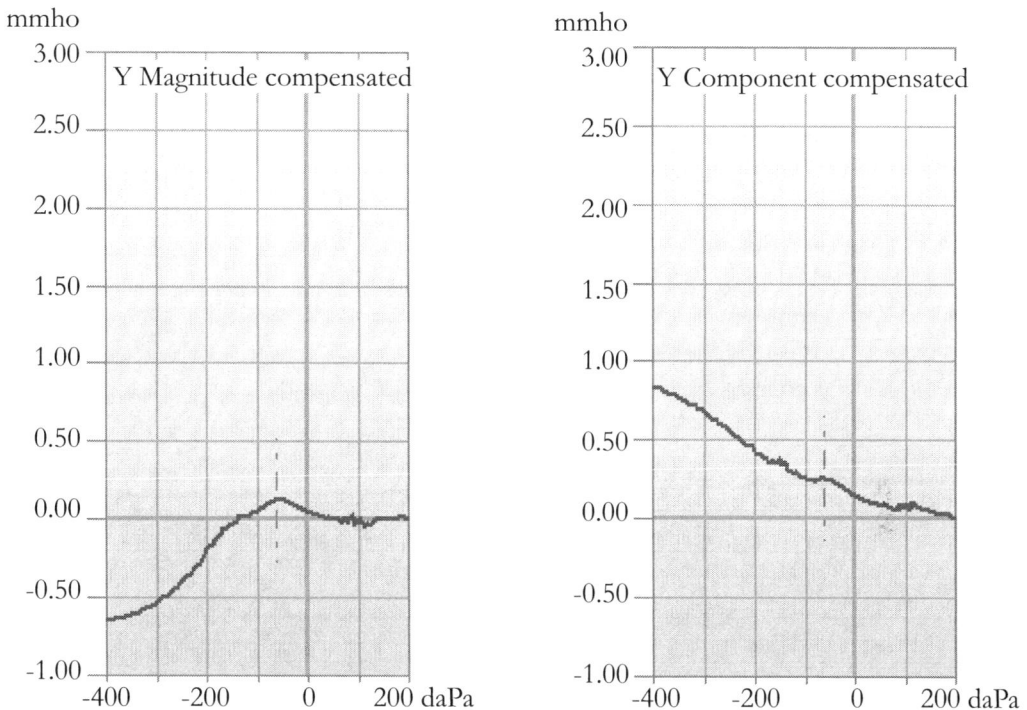

FIGURE 3–11. Tympanograms obtained from the left ear of a 3-day-old female (RM), who passed the AABR, TEOAE, and ASR tests. The HFT results show a shallow positive peak, with peak compensated static admittance values falling below the 5th percentile of the normative data. Despite this apparently abnormal HFT finding, there is no obvious concern about the middle ear function in RM's ear.

Case 7

The baby, JT, was a male with gestational age 39 weeks and birth weight 3.8 kg. The birth was uneventful. He passed the newborn hearing screening conducted by Queensland Health. He was tested when he was 2 days old. During the test, he was asleep but restless at times. He had robust TEOAEs (SNRs were 8, 17, 24, 17, and 17 dB at 1, 1.5, 2, 3, and 4 kHz, respectively) in his right ear. Ipsilateral acoustic stapedial reflex thresholds for the 2 kHz and BBN stimuli were 75 and 55 dB HL, respectively. His HFT results, shown in Fig-

ure 3–12, indicate negative magnitude compensated static admittance with no identifiable peak. The component compensated tympanogram showed positive component compensated static admittance with no identifiable peak. These patterns of HFT results would be regarded as abnormal findings according to the pass criteria for HFT. However, given that JT has passed the AABR screening, and TEOAE and ASR tests, he should have normal auditory function up to the brainstem region. The HFT findings, being inconsistent with other test results, may be regarded as false positive results. A longitudinal study to

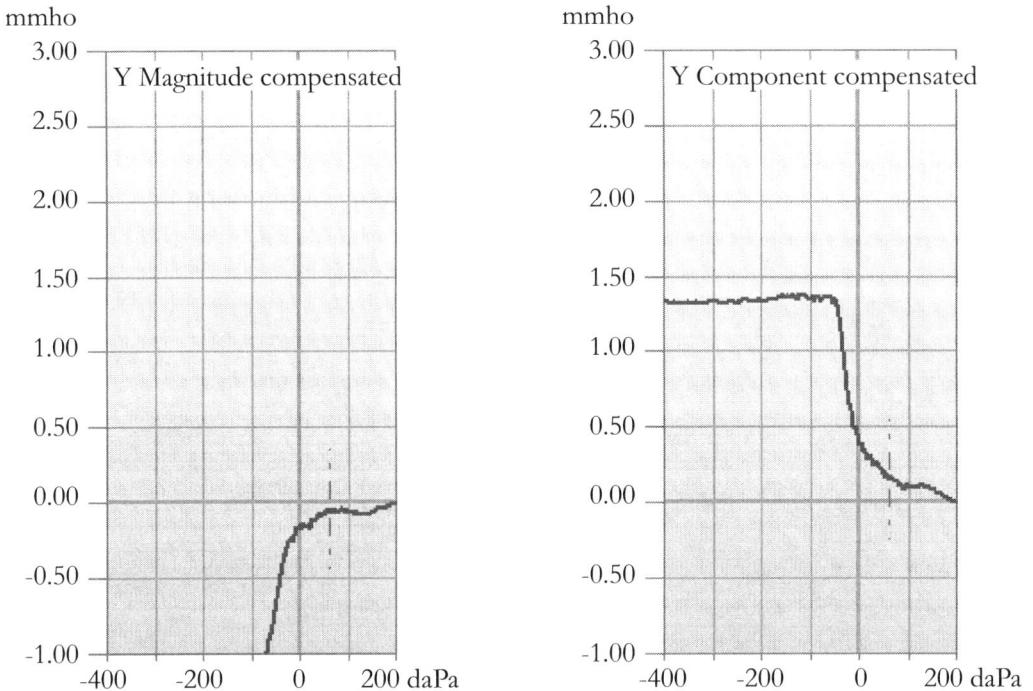

FIGURE 3–12. Tympanograms obtained from the right ear of a 2-day-old male (JT), who passed the AABR, TEOAE, and ASR tests. The HFT results show negative magnitude compensated static admittance with no identifiable peak. The corresponding component compensated static admittance tympanogram indicates abnormal findings. The HFT findings, being inconsistent with other test results, may be regarded as false-positive results.

check the development of the HFT findings in this case would be beneficial.

Case 8

The baby, CM, was a male with gestational age 41.4 weeks and birth weight 4.0 kg. He passed the newborn hearing screening. He was tested at 34 hours after birth. Although he slept during the test, he was a bit restless and required a pacifier. His left ear exhibited robust TEOAEs (SNRs were 6, 11, 24, 20, and 28 dB at 1, 1.5, 2, 3, and 4 kHz, respectively). Ipsilateral acoustic stapedial reflex thresholds for the 2 kHz and BBN stimuli were 75 and 65 dB HL, respectively. His HFT results, shown in Figure 3–13, indicated a flat response from +200 to −70 daPa and then dropped sharply as the pressure is decreased to −400 daPa. The component compensated tympanogram showed no identifiable peak with component compensated static admittance increasing linearly from 0 mmho at +40 daPa to 1 mmho at −200 daPa. These patterns of HFT results would have been regarded as abnormal findings. However, given

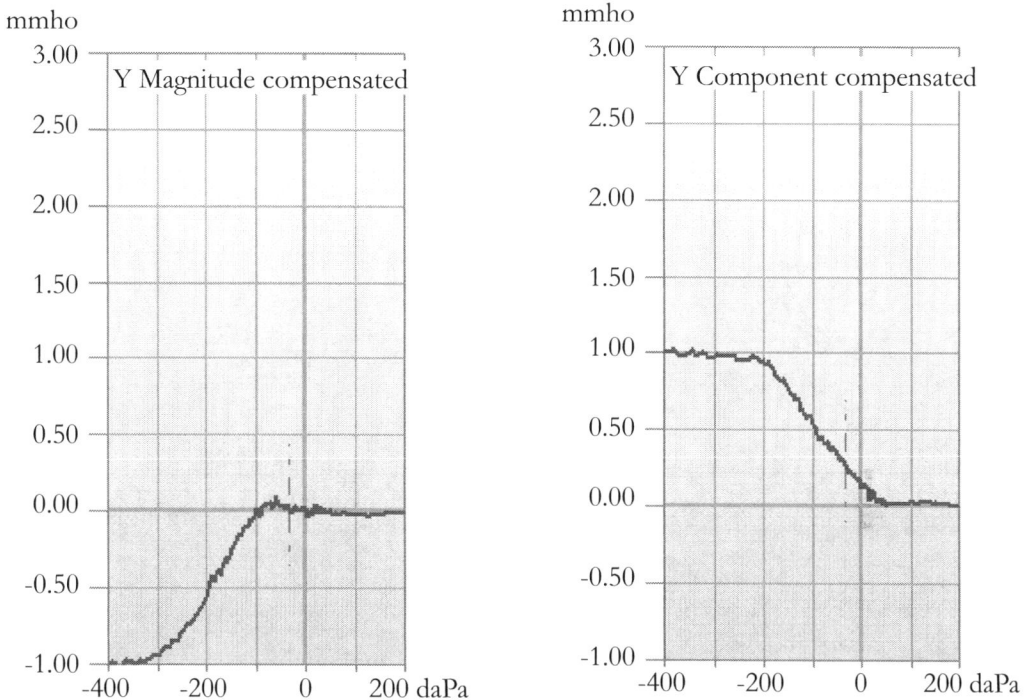

FIGURE 3–13. Tympanograms obtained from the left ear of a 34-hour-old male (CM), who passed the AABR, TEOAE, and ASR tests. His magnitude compensated tympanogram indicates a flat response from +200 to –70 daPa with no identifiable peak. The component compensated tympanogram shows no identifiable peak either. The HFT findings, being inconsistent with other test results, may be regarded as false-positive results. This case illustrates the importance of a test battery approach to evaluating the auditory function of neonates.

that CM passed the AABR screening, and TEOAE and ASR tests, he should have normal auditory function up to the brainstem region. In this special case, the HFT findings may be regarded as abnormal. At the very least, the HFT findings were inconclusive.

Case 9

The baby, AN, was a female with gestational age 38.6 weeks and birth weight 2.9 kg. She passed the newborn hearing screening. She was tested 2 days after birth and was asleep during the test. Her left ear showed robust TEOAEs (SNRs were 0, 22, 25, 25, and 29 dB at 1, 1.5, 2, 3, and 4 kHz, respectively). Ipsilateral acoustic stapedial reflex thresholds for the 2 kHz and BBN stimuli were 65 and 60 dB HL, respectively. The magnitude and component compensated tympanograms, shown in Figure 3–14, were similar in shape to those of the previous case (Case 8). Although a very shallow

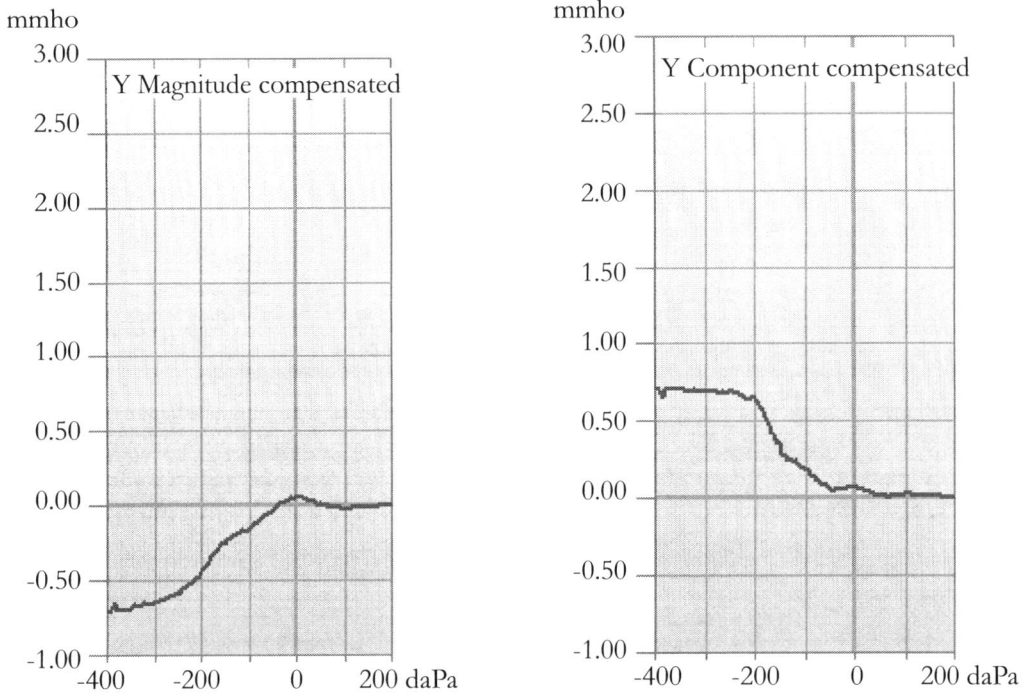

FIGURE 3–14. Tympanograms obtained from the left ear of a 2-day-old female (AN), who passed the AABR, TEOAE, and ASR tests. The magnitude and component compensated tympanograms show a very shallow peak at 0 daPa. However, these results did not qualify for a pass in HFT due to inadequate seal of the probe tip.

peak at 0 daPa was identified in the tympanograms, these results would be regarded as borderline abnormal findings. However, given that AN passed the AABR screening, and TEOAE and ASR tests, she should have normal auditory function up to the brainstem region. In view of this apparent discrepancy with expected normal results, the HFT test was repeated with due attention paid to acquiring a snugly fitted probe seal. The retest results, shown in Figure 3–15, revealed normal HFT findings with magnitude compensated static admittance of 1.05 mmho and component compensated static

admittance of 1.38 mmho at 25 daPa TPP. This special case illustrates the importance of having an adequate seal in HFT testing and that retest is necessary especially when unexpected results occur.

REFERENCES

Alaerts, J., Luts, H., & Wouters, J. (2007). Evaluation of middle ear function in young children: Clinical guidelines for the use of 226- and 1000-Hz tympanometry. *Otology and Neurotology, 28,* 727–732.

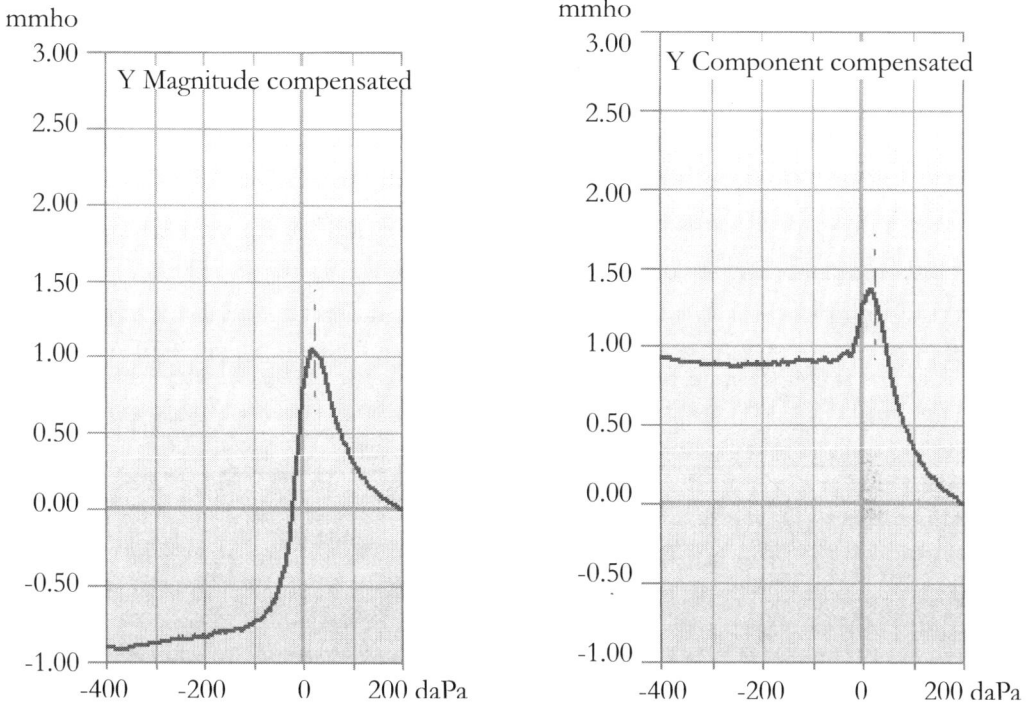

FIGURE 3–15. Tympanograms obtained from the same neonate (AN) in a second attempt with a snugly fitted probe tip. The retest results revealed normal HFT findings. This case illustrates the importance of having an adequate seal in HFT testing.

American National Standards Institute. (ANSI). (1987). *Specifications for instruments to measure aural acoustic impedance and admittance (aural acoustic immittance)*. ANSI S3.39-1987. New York, NY: Author.

Baldwin, M. (2006). Choice of probe tone and classification of trace patterns in tympanometry undertaken in early infancy. *International Journal of Audiology, 45*, 417–427.

Bluestone, C., Beery, Q., & Paradise, J. L. (1973). Audiometry and tympanometry in relation to middle ear effusions in children. *Laryngoscope, 83*, 594–604.

Boswell, J., & Nienhuys, T. (1995). Onset of otitis media in the first eight weeks of life in Aboriginal and non-Aboriginal Australians. *Annals of Otology, Rhinology, and Laryngology, 104*, 542–549.

Calandruccio, L., Fitzgerald, T. S., & Prieve, B. A. (2006). Normative multifrequency tympanometry in infants and toddlers. *Journal of the American Academy of Audiology, 17*, 470–480.

Cantekin, E. I., Bluestone, C. D., Fria, T. J., Stool, S. E., Beery, Q. C., & Sabo, D. L. (1980). Identification of otitis media with effusion in children. *Annals of Otology, Rhinology, and Laryngology, 89*(Suppl. 68), 190–195.

Jerger, J. (1970). Clinical experience with impedance audiometry. *Archives of Otolaryngology, 92*, 311–324.

Joint Committee on Infant Hearing (JCIH). (2007). Year 2007 position statement: Principles and guidelines for early detection and intervention programs. *Pediatrics, 120,* 898–921.

Kei, J., Allison-Levrick, J., Dockray, J., Harrys, R., Kirkegard, C., Wong, J., . . . Tudehope, D. (2003). High frequency (1000 Hz) tympanometry in normal neonates. *Journal of the American Academy of Audiology, 14,* 20–28.

Kei, J., Mazlan, R., Hickson, L., Gavranich, J., & Linning, R. (2007). Measuring middle ear admittance in newborns using 1000 Hz tympanometry: A comparison of methodologies. *Journal of the American Academy of Audiology, 18,* 739–748.

Marchant, C. D., McMillan, P. M., Shurin, P. A., Johnson, C. E., Turczyk, R. N., Feinstein, J. C., & Panek, D. M. (1986). Objective diagnosis of otitis media in early infancy by tympanometry and ipsilateral acoustic reflex thresholds. *Journal of Pediatrics, 109,* 590–595.

Margolis, R. H., Bass-Ringdahl, S., Hanks, W. D., Holte, L., & Zapala, D. A. (2003). Tympanometry in newborn infants—1 kHz norms. *Journal of the American Academy of Audiology, 14,* 383–391.

Margolis, R. H., & Hunter, L. L. (2000). Acoustic immittance measurements. In R. J. Roeser, M. Valente & H. Hosford-Dunn (Eds.), *Audiology diagnosis.* New York, NY: Thieme.

Margolis, R. H., & Smith, P. (1977). Tympanometric asymmetry. *Journal of Speech and Hearing Research, 20,* 437–446.

Mazlan, R., Kei, J., & Hickson, L. (2009a). Test-retest reliability of acoustic reflex testing in healthy newborns. *Ear and Hearing, 30,* 295–301.

Mazlan, R., Kei, J., Hickson, L., Gavranich, J., & Linning, R. (2009b). High frequency (1000 Hz) tympanometry findings in newborns: Normative data using a compo-nent compensated admittance approach. *Australian and New Zealand Journal of Audiology, 31,* 15–24.

Mazlan, R., Kei, J., Hickson, L., Stapleton, C., Grant, S., Lim, S., . . . Linning, R. (2007). High frequency immittance findings: Newborn versus 6-week-old infants. *International Journal of Audiology, 46,* 711–717.

Purdy, S., & Williams, M. J. (2000). High frequency tympanometry: A valid and reliable immittance test protocol for young infants? *New Zealand Audiological Society Bulletin, 10,* 9–24.

Queensland Health. (2007). *Healthy Hearing Program—A statewide universal neonatal hearing screening program.* Retrieved on 24 September, 2010 from http://www.health.qld.gov.au/healthy hearing/docs/background.pdf

Rabinowitz, W. (1981).Measurement of the acoustic input immittance of the human ear. *Journal of the Acoustical Society of America, 70,* 1025–1035.

Rhodes, M. C., Margolis, R. H., Hirsch, J. E., & Napp, A. P. (1999). Hearing screening in the newborn intensive care nursery: Comparison of methods. *Otolaryngology-Head and Neck Surgery, 120,* 799–808.

Shanks J. (1984).Tympanometry. *Ear and Hearing, 5,* 268–280.

Shanks, J., & Lily, D. (1981). An evaluation of tympanometric estimates of ear canal volume. *Journal of Speech and Hearing Research, 24,* 557–566.

Swanepoel, D. W., Werner, S., Hugo, R., Louw, B., Owen, R., & Swanepoel, A. (2007). High frequency immittance for neonates: A normative study. *Acta Otolaryngologica, 127,* 49–56.

Terkildsen, K., & Thompsen, K.A. (1959). The influence of pressure variations on the impedance of the human ear drum. *Journal of Laryngology and Otology, 73,* 409–418.

Vanhuyse, V. J., Creten, W. L., & Van Camp, K. J. (1975). On the W-notching of tympanogram. *Scandinavian Audiology, 4*, 45–50.

Vanpeperstraete, V., Creten, W., & Van Camp, K. (1979). On the asymmetry of susceptance tympanograms. *Scandinavian Audiology, 8*, 173–179.

Williams, M. J., Purdy, S. C., & Barber, C. S. (1995). High frequency probe tone tympanometry in infants with middle ear effusion. *Australian Journal of Otolaryngology, 2*, 169–173.

CHAPTER 4

Acoustic Stapedial Reflexes: Clinical Applications

JOSEPH KEI AND RAFIDAH MAZLAN

INTRODUCTION

The acoustic stapedial reflex (ASR) is a reflexive contraction of the stapedius muscle of the middle ear in response to a loud sound presented to a healthy ear. The ASR test is usually performed following tympanometry to assess the function of the ear up to the brainstem region. The ASR test together with pure tone audiometry, tympanometry and speech audiometry form a basic battery of tests in an audiology clinic. It has wide clinical applications in identifying auditory dysfunction in humans. Although the ASR test is routinely used in a diagnostic test battery for adults, it is not commonly used with young infants at present.

This chapter provides an outline of the principles of the ASR with particular emphasis on its clinical application to young infants. Recent research findings on normative ASR data and test-retest reliability of the ASR threshold obtained from young infants are presented. The chapter concludes with case reports illustrating the application of ASR in conjunction with the automated auditory brainstem response, transient evoked otoacoustic emissions, and high frequency tympanometry tests to assess the auditory function of young infants.

PRINCIPLES OF THE ACOUSTIC STAPEDIAL REFLEX (ASR)

The ASR test involves the presentation of a pure tone signal or noise stimulus to elicit a reflex response from the stapedius muscle in the middle ear. The neural network of the stapedial reflex is located in the lower brainstem and consists of both ipsilateral and contralateral routes. Activation of the stapedial muscle, involves three to four neurons for the ipsilateral route and four neurons for the contralateral route. When an intense acoustic stimulus is presented to a normal auditory system, the stapedius muscle which is attached to the head of the stapes, will contract in response to the stimulation (Gelfand, 2009). When the muscle contracts, the stapes is pulled away from the oval window and the ossicular chain stiffens. Hence, the contraction of the stapedius muscle changes the mechanical properties of the middle ear by altering the amount of sound energy going into the middle ear system. In conventional tympanometry using a 226-Hz probe tone, contraction of the stapedial muscle is consistent with an increase in the impedance of the middle ear system which is reflected as a decrease in admittance. This decrease in admittance, which is seen as an increase in stiffness of the ossicular chain, generally has been accepted as an ASR response.

In normal ears, the ASR is a bilateral phenomenon where the muscles in both ears contract in response to an adequate acoustic stimulus presented to either ear. There are two ways of eliciting an ASR: (1) by ipsilateral stimulation, or (2) by contralateral stimulation. In ipsilateral stimulation, the eliciting signal is presented to the same ear in which acoustic immittance changes are being measured, whereas contralateral stimulation involves presenting the eliciting signal to one ear (usually referred to as the stimulus ear) and measuring the acoustic immittance changes in the opposite ear (the probe ear).

In a diagnostic ASR test, it is common to measure the ASR threshold (ASRT) using both the ipsilateral and contralateral stimulation methods. The ASRT is defined as the lowest stimulus intensity level that produces a just detectable change in acoustic admittance as a result of the contraction of the stapedius muscle (Northern & Downs, 2001). The activating stimuli are usually pure tones of 0.5, 1, 2, and 4 kHz. Some clinicians do not test ASR at 4 kHz as ASRT may be elevated or ASR not present in normally hearing young adults due possibly to rapid adaptation at this frequency (Gelfand 1984; Silman & Silverman, 1991). In some cases, the ASRT of a broadband noise (BBN) stimulus is also measured. Using the Sensitivity Prediction with the Acoustic Reflex test, it is possible to estimate the degree of hearing loss based on the difference in ASRT between the BBN and pure-tone activators (0.5, 1, and 2 kHz) (Jerger, Anthony, Jerger, & Mauldin, 1974a; Jerger, Hayes, Anthony, & Mauldin, 1978).

In essence, the integrity of the ASR pathway (the peripheral auditory system up to the brainstem region) can be evaluated. The diagnostic applications of the ASR include estimation of hearing levels (Hall, 1978; Jerger et al., 1974a; Niemeyer & Sesterhenn, 1974), site of lesion testing to diagnose conductive, cochlear and retrocochlear pathologies (Ferguson, Smith, Lutman, Mason, Coles, & Gibbin, 1996; Handler & Margolis, 1977; Jerger, Burney, Mauldin, & Crump, 1974b), evaluation of facial nerve dysfunction (Alford, Jerger, Coats, Peterson, & Weber, 1973; Citron & Adour, 1978), and confirmation of functional or nonorganic hearing loss (Gelfand, 1994). Any abnormal findings such as raised ASRTs or absent ASRs would alert clinicians to suspect disorders in the auditory pathway. Despite its clinical significance, the ASR test, to date, has not been widely applied to young infants (0 to 6 months).

Acoustic Stapedial Reflex Patterns in Newborns and Young Infants

Weatherby and Bennett (1980) found that ASRs are present in healthy neonates when the probe-tone frequency was increased to 800 Hz or higher. However, at these high probe tone frequencies, the chance of getting an upward reflex (increase in admittance) in the ASR results is increased. The increase in admittance is partly caused by a functional decoupling of the stapes from the cochlea (Borg, 1968; Moller, 1961), thus limiting sound energy being transmitted into the cochlea. Bennett and Weatherby (1979), in a study investigating the effect of multiple probe frequency (220 to 2000 Hz) on ASR in normally hearing adults, found that the direction of change of impedance (the reciprocal of admittance) is dependent on the probe tone frequency. They found that the ASR increases the middle ear impedance for probe tones of frequencies up to 700 Hz, and decreases it for higher frequencies.

Weatherby and Bennett (1980), and Bennett and Weatherby (1982) have shown that the reflex pattern (direction

of change of impedance) can shift in adults and newborns as a function of the probe tone frequency. Weatherby and Bennett (1980) show that the probe tone frequency at which the reflex pattern shifts is considerably higher in newborns (1200 Hz) than in adults (665 Hz). The shift occurs due to reduction of both resistance and reactance at higher probe-tone frequency (closer to the resonance frequency of the middle ear) which will result in a decrease in the impedance (increase in the admittance) and be observed as a deflection or upward movement in reflex tracing. Mazlan, Kei, and Hickson (2009) found that 4% of the neonatal ears showed an upward reflex when stimulated by a 2-kHz pure tone and BBN stimuli. Kei (in press) found that the upward reflex pattern was present in 32.4%, 20.6%, 23.5%, and 11.8% of 68 ears stimulated by the 0.5 kHz, 2 kHz, 4 kHz, and BBN, respectively.

An example of an upward reflex pattern obtained from a 2-day-old female is shown in Figure 4–1. Her ASR results at 2 kHz clearly show a growth in the reflex magnitude as the stimulus intensity increased from 65 to 75 dB HL. This upward reflex pattern cannot be regarded as an artifact because an artifact may not be repeatable and does not necessarily grow with increasing stimulus intensity.

Normative ASR Data in Young Infants

Swanepoel, Werner, Hugo, Louw, Owen, and Swanepoel (2007) and Mazlan et al.

Deflection, Ipsi 2000 Hz

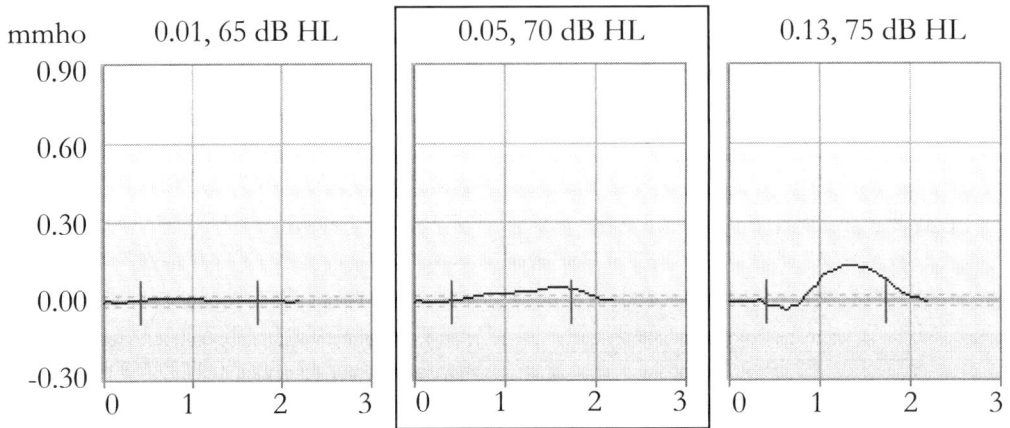

FIGURE 4–1. ASR results obtained from a 2-day-old female using a probe tone of 1 kHz and stimulated ipsilaterally by a 2-kHz tone. An upward reflex pattern was found showing a growth in the reflex magnitude as the stimulus intensity increased from 65 to 75 dB HL.

(2007) investigated the use of the ASR test with young infants. The ASRTs were determined when an admittance change exceeded 0.02 mmho. The percentage presence of ASR in normal neonates was reported to be 94% and 100% for Swanepoel et al. (2007)and Mazlan et al. (2007) studies, respectively. These findings indicate that ASR is generally present in healthy newborns and young infants.

Mazlan et al. (2007) successfully recorded ipsilateral ASRs in all 41 neonates with a mean chronological age of 61.7 hours (SD = 42.7 hours) using a probe tone of 1 kHz and activating stimuli of a 2-kHz tone and BBN. The mean ASRT for the 2-kHz tone was 73 dB HL (SD = 10 dB), whereas that for the BBN was 59 dB HL (SD = 10 dB). As the stimulus intensity of the tympanometer could not go below 50 dB HL, the ASRT

for some neonates could not be established. For these neonates, an ASRT value of 50 dB HL was assigned. Hence, the mean ASRT for the BBN could have been overestimated.

In another study, Mazlan and colleagues (2009) measured ASRT in 194 neonates. They obtained an average ASRT of 76 dB HL (SD = 8 dB) for the 2-kHz stimulus. However, the mean ASRT of 65 dB HL (SD = 8 dB) for the BBN was overestimated as Mazlan et al. (2009) excluded data with ASRTs of 50 dB HL from their analysis.

Kei (in press) conducted a normative ASR study which incorporated stimulating tones of 0.5 and 4 kHz in addition to the 2-kHz tone and BBN. Sixty-eight neonates, who passed AABR, TEOAE and HFT tests, participated in the study. These babies were born full-term with a mean gestational age of

39.6 weeks (range = 37 to 42 weeks). Their chronological age ranged from 1 to 16 days (mean = 2.5 days, SD = 1.8 days). Their mean birth weight was 3.5 kg (SD = 0.6 kg). The inclusion criteria were: normal birth history within the first 24 hours, no congenital defects, a normal maternal history and pregnancy, and no historical or hereditary risk factors. Risk factors resulting in exclusion from the study were those outlined by the Joint Committee on Infant Hearing (JCIH, 2007). The normative ASRT data are shown in Table 4–1 alongside the data from Mazlan et al. (2007) and Mazlan et al. (2009) for comparison. Kei (in press) revealed that the mean ASRT for the 0.5-kHz tone was significantly greater than that for the 2 kHz tone, which in turn was significantly greater than that for the 4-kHz tone. It can be deduced from the normative data that the ASRTs should not exceed 95, 85, 80, and 75 dB HL for the 0.5, 2, 4 kHz, and BBN, respectively, to be considered normal ASR results for neonates.

Normative ASR data for other age groups are scarce. Preliminary findings from the Mazlan et al. (2007) study showed an increase in mean ASRT for the 2 kHz stimulus from 73 dB for the newborns to 80 dB HL for 6-week-old infants. The increase in ASRT may be caused by an increase in size of the neonates' external ear canal and changes in the vibratory motion of external auditory canal walls in response to acoustic stimuli (Holte, Margolis, & Cavanaugh, 1991). For the BBN stimulus, the trend of increasing mean ASRT with age is apparent (Mazlan et al., 2007).

Suggested ASR Protocol for Testing Young Infants

Although a comprehensive ASR testing procedure including both ipsilateral and contralateral stimulations is ideal for a wide range of diagnostic applications, it is not commonly performed on young infants. In general, ipsilateral ASRT results are adequate for general

TABLE 4–1. Mean ± SD and 90% Range of Ipsilateral Acoustic Stapedial Reflex Thresholds, Elicited by Broadband Noise (BBN) and Pure-Tone Stimuli from Neonates in Three Studies

Study	N (ears)	0.5 kHz	2 kHz	4 kHz	BBN
Mazlan et al. (2007)	41		73 ± 10 dB (50–90 dB)		NA (50–85 dB)
Mazlan et al. (2009)	194		76 ± 8 dB (65–90 dB)		NA (50–80 dB)
Kei (in press)	68	82 ± 8 dB (70–95 dB)	71 ± 8 dB (60–85 dB)	65 ± 9 dB (50–80 dB)	NA (50–75 dB)

NA means not applicable.

diagnostic purposes, although contralateral ASR testing may provide useful clinical information for detecting intra-axial brainstem lesions. Furthermore, acquiring contralateral ASRTs in young infants requires a long testing time. In fact, acquiring ASRTs from neonates by contralateral stimulation is a more demanding task than from adults because of the need to maintain a good probe seal in both ears.

In the context of assessing middle ear function in young infants, ipsilateral stimulation offers advantages over contralateral testing. First, ipsilateral ASRs are sensitive to middle ear pathology. Numerous studies have demonstrated that absent or elevated ipsilateral reflexes were closely associated with middle ear effusion (Geddes, 1987; Hirsch, Margolis, & Rykken, 1992; Marchant, McMillan, Shurin, Johnson, Turczyk, Feinstein, & Panek, 1986; Nozza, Bluestone, Kardatzke, & Bachman, 1992). Second, ipsilateral testing eliminates the confusion of which ear is being tested and results obtained from ipsilateral testing are not influenced by disorders that affect the contralateral ear. Third, the procedure involved during ipsilateral testing is easier and more feasible for neonates and infants as it does not involve placing another earphone on the opposite ear as required in contralateral testing (Gelfand, 2009). Finally, a higher percentage of ASR presence may be obtained with ipsilateral stimulation than with contralateral stimulation (McMillan, Bennett, Marchant, & Shurin, 1985). On the other hand, ipsilateral stimulation with an activating stimulus (e.g., 1 kHz) having the same frequency as the probe tone (1 kHz) can be problematic because of the possible acoustic interaction between the probe tone and activating tone.

The intensity level of the probe tone should not be too high as to elicit an ASR or behavioral response from a young infant (0 to 6 months). Given the small ear canal volume of a young infant, a probe tone of 1 kHz delivered to the ear at 85 dB SPL may be excessive. In particular, such high intensity level probe tone may affect the measurement of ASRT especially in the ipsilateral stimulation mode. Hence, to reduce the impact of a high intensity level probe tone on ASRT, a lower level such as 75 dB SPL is recommended when testing young infants (Mazlan et al., 2009).

Diagnostic evaluation of auditory function in young infants using ASR should include stimuli of various frequencies. Although it is not advisable to use a 1-kHz activating tone, other tones such as 0.5, 2, and 4 kHz may be utilized. Kei (in press) found that ASRs were present in healthy neonates at these frequencies, with mean ASRT at 4 kHz being significantly smaller than that at other frequencies. This finding is in stark contrast with ASR results for normally hearing adults who may exhibit elevated ASRT or absent ASR at 4 kHz (Gelfand 1984; Silman & Silverman, 1991). Hence, testing ASR at 4 kHz in young infants has the advantages of getting a frequency-specific response at this high frequency, eliciting an ASR response at a lower level which is unlikely to evoke an uncomfortable behavioral response.

As regards the method used to elicit an ASR response, either the manual or autosearch method is suitable. Using a manual searching method, an activating stimulus is initially presented at 70 dB HL for one second to the ear. If no response is observed, the stimulus level is increased in 5 dB steps until a response is obtained or a maximum level of 105 dB is reached. ASRT is defined as the lowest intensity at which a change in admittance of 0.02 mmho is detected. The change in admittance can be an increase (upward reflex pattern) or decrease (downward reflex pattern) in admittance compared to the baseline. Alternatively, a criterion change of admittance of 0.03 or 0.04 mmho may be used. Regardless of what criterion admittance value is used, it is important to check for repeatability of the ASR response.

The autosearch method, available from the Masen Otoflex 100 device, employs a programmed protocol in detecting an ASR. The tester can program the testing procedure by testing ASR in a pre-determined sequence of the stimuli (e.g., 4 kHz, 2 kHz, and 0.5 kHz). The stimulus is presented initially at an intensity level of 70 dB HL for 1 second. If an ASR response is elicited at this level, the intensity will be decreased in 5-dB steps until the ASR disappears (e.g., change in admittance is smaller than a criterion value of 0.02 mmho). When this happens, the device will increase the intensity level by 5 dB to elicit an ASR response to ensure repeatability. This stimulus level is then recorded by the device as the ASRT for this stimulus. If, however, an ASR response is not elicited at an initial presentation level of 70 dB HL, the intensity level will be increased in 5-dB steps until an ASR is elicited or when the maximum output (105 dB HL) is reached. In this ascending process, when an ASR is first detected at a certain stimulus level, the device will increase the stimulus level by 5 dB to evoke an ASR with a greater change in admittance. When this happens, the previous stimulus level will be taken as the ASRT. In confirming an ASR response, it is essential to confirm that the change in admittance (in either direction) increases with stimulus intensity beyond the threshold level. An artefact or behavioral response will be suspected otherwise.

The activity of young infants during the ASR test may affect the accuracy of the ASRT measurement. Unlike adults, young infants do not usually stay still during the ASR test. Hence, some precautions should be taken when conducting the ASR test on young infants. It is better to test the infant when he/she is asleep after a feed. Whenever possible, ask an assistant to observe the activity of the infant so that the change in admittance does not synchronize with the infant's jaw or limb movement. If the infant is awake and restless with mild activity (such as irregular respiration, movements of one or more limbs or head, some eye or facial movement), testing should be stopped (Keith & Bench, 1978). When a high stimulus level (>90 dB HL) is used, the infant may be disturbed resulting in a behavioral response (e.g., infant may stir, blink his/her eyes or even startle) which may produce a sudden change in admittance in synchrony with the stimulus. When this happens, the ASR results are invalid.

CASE STUDIES ILLUSTRATING THE APPLICATIONS OF THE ASR TEST

The cases reported in this section are babies assessed between 2009 and 2010. The purpose for showing these cases is to illustrate the application of the ASR test when used in conjunction with other tests such as the AABR, TEOAE, and HFT tests. In the case studies described below, only one ear was tested. The pass criteria for the TEOAE and HFT tests are the same as those described in Chapter 3. Briefly, the pass criterion for the TEOAE test was a 3 dB or greater signal-to-noise ratio (SNR) in at least four out of five half-octave bands centered at 1, 1.5, 2, 3, and 4 kHz (Mazlan et al., 2009). The pass criterion for the HFT test was a single positive-peaked admittance tympanogram with either a magnitude compensated static admittance of at least 0.2 mmho or a component compensated static admittance of at least 0.4 mmho (Mazlan et al., 2009). As for the ASR test, a pass was awarded if the ipsilateral ASRT was less than 100, 95, 90, and 85 dB HL for the 0.5-, 2-, and 4-kHz tone, and broadband noise (BBN) stimuli, respectively.

Case 1

Baby boy, TS, was born at 39 weeks of gestation with a birth weight of 2.9 kg. The birth was uneventful. He passed the AABR screening test conducted by Queensland Health nurses. He was 3 days old at time of assessment and was asleep during the test. TEOAEs were present at normal levels in the left ear (SNR = −1, 3, 16, 24, and 18 dB at 1, 1.5, 2, 3, and 4 kHz, respectively). Ipsilateral acoustic stapedial reflexes were present at normal threshold levels (ASRT = 80, 70, 75, and 50 dB HL for 0.5 kHz, 2 kHz, 4 kHz, and BBN, respectively). An upward reflex pattern was observed for all stimuli of the ASR test except for 4 kHz. Figure 4–2 shows some of the ASR findings which include ASRTs of 80 and 50 dB HL at 0.5 kHz and BBN, respectively. The magnitude compensated tympanogram shows a single peak with middle ear admittance of 0.95 mmho at a tympanometric peak pressure (TPP) of 55 daPa. Taken together, baby TS's test results are consistent with normal auditory function up to the brainstem region.

Case 2

Baby boy, VL, was born at 38 weeks of gestation with a birth weight of 2.2 kg. He was one of the twins and was in Neonatal Intensive Care Unit for 5 days. He was 5 days old at the time of assessment. During the test, he was awake and peaceful but required a dummy at times. He passed the AABR screening test. TEOAEs were just adequate to be awarded a pass in his right ear (SNR = −5, 3, 3, 5, and 6 dB at 1, 1.5, 2, 3, and 4 kHz, respectively). Ipsilateral ASRs were present at normal threshold levels (80, 65, 80, and 75 dB HL for 0.5 kHz, 2 kHz, 4 kHz, and BBN, respectively). Figure 4–3 shows some of the ASR findings which include ASRTs of 65 and 80 dB HL at 2 and 4 kHz, respectively.

Deflection, Ipsi 500 Hz

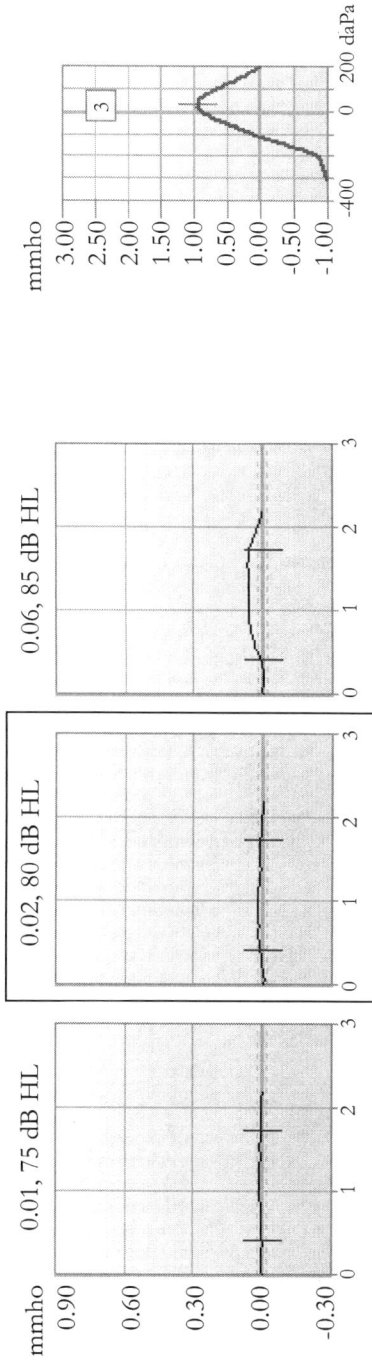

mmho

0.90 — 0.60 — 0.30 — 0.00 — -0.30

0.01, 75 dB HL   0.02, 80 dB HL   0.06, 85 dB HL

Deflection, Ipsi BBN

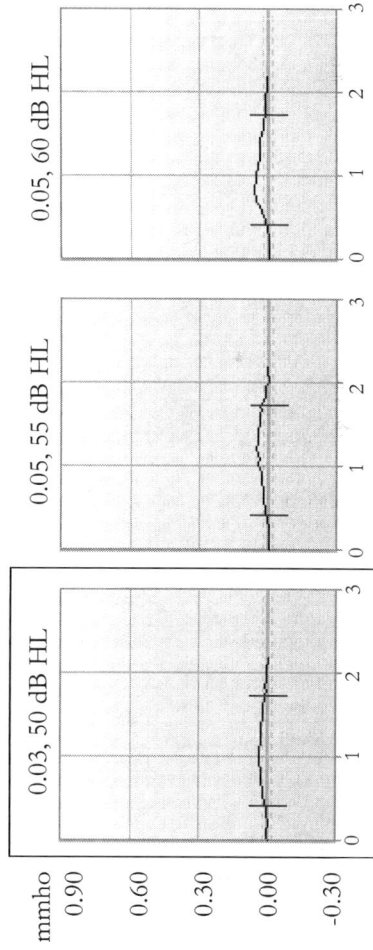

mmho

0.90 — 0.60 — 0.30 — 0.00 — -0.30

0.03, 50 dB HL   0.05, 55 dB HL   0.05, 60 dB HL

mmho

3.00 — 2.50 — 2.00 — 1.50 — 1.00 — 0.50 — 0.00 — -0.50 — -1.00

3

-400   0   200 daPa

FIGURE 4–2. ASR findings obtained from a 3-day-old male (TS) who passed the AABR, TEOAE, and HFT tests in his left ear. The results revealed ASRTs of 80 and 50 dB HL at 0.5 kHz and BBN, respectively. The magnitude compensated tympanogram shows a single peak with middle ear admittance of 0.95 mmho at a TPP of 55 daPa.

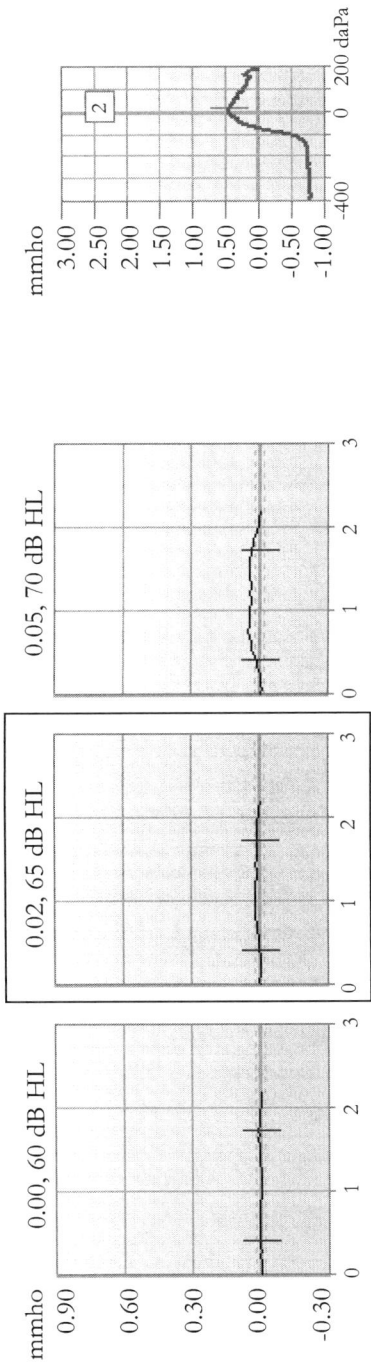

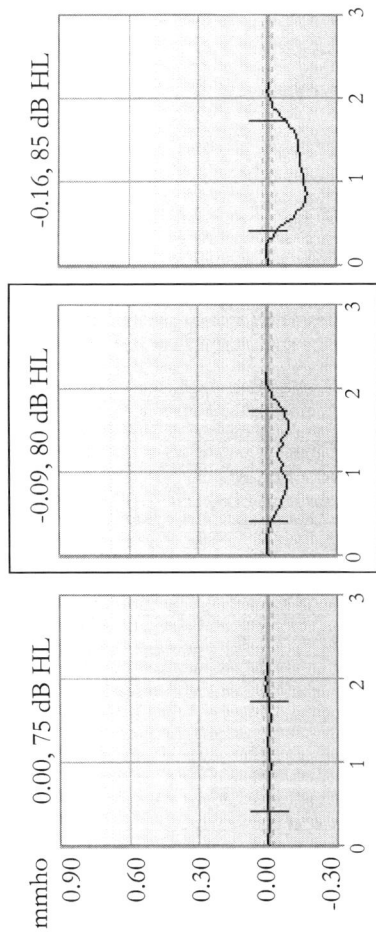

FIGURE 4–3. ASR findings obtained from a 5-day-old male (VL) who passed the AABR, TEOAE, and HFT tests in his right ear. The results revealed ASRTs of 65 and 80 dB HL at 2 and 4 kHz, respectively. The magnitude compensated tympanogram shows a single peak with middle ear admittance of 0.4 mmho at a TPP of 30 daPa.

Upward reflexes were observed for the 2 kHz stimulus only. The magnitude compensated tympanogram shows a middle ear admittance of 0.4 mmho at a TPP of 30 daPa. Despite the weak TEOAEs, baby VL's test results indicate normal auditory function up to the brainstem region.

Case 3

Baby girl, LT, was born at 39 weeks of gestation with a birth weight of 3.7 kg. She was 2 days old and was asleep at the time of assessment. She passed the AABR screening test, but failed the TEOAE test with no emissions recorded from 1 to 4 kHz in the left ear. Based on the AABR and TEOAE results, the possibility of a slight to mild conductive or cochlear hearing loss cannot be excluded. Further testing using HFT indicated a normal tympanogram with a magnitude compensated admittance of 1.2 mmho at a TPP of 90 daPa as shown in Figure 4–4. Interestingly, ipsilateral ASRs were present at normal threshold levels (95, 75, 75, and 75 dB HL for the 0.5 kHz, 2 kHz, 4 kHz, and BBN, respectively) with upward reflexes observed at 0.5 and 4 kHz (as shown). The presence of ASR at normal levels indicates that middle ear dysfunction was unlikely to be the cause of the hearing loss. Nevertheless, the presence of normal ASRT cannot exclude the possibility of a mild cochlear hearing loss because of the loudness recruitment effect. In conclusion, all of the above results are consistent with a mild cochlear hearing loss in the left ear. Further investigations using tone-burst

ABR or auditory steady-state response (ASSR) would be required to ascertain the degree of hearing loss for LT.

Case 4

Baby boy, KS, was born at 39 weeks of gestation with a birth weight of 3.3 kg. He was 2 days old at the time of assessment. During the test, he was asleep. He passed the AABR screening test. TEOAEs were present at normal levels in his left ear. His HFT results, shown in Figure 4–5, indicate normal findings (TPP = 60 daPa; magnitude compensated admittance = 0.48 mmho; component compensated admittance = 1.3 mmho). Surprisingly, ipsilateral ASRs were absent. Taken together, these results are not consistent with normal auditory function. Further audiological assessments using ABR and ASSR are required to ascertain the hearing function of KS.

Case 5

Baby boy, MJ, was born at 39.9 weeks of gestation with a birth weight of 2.8 kg. He was 2 days old at the time of assessment. During the test, he was asleep. He passed the AABR screen, but failed in the TEOAE test in the right ear. These results suggest the possibility of either a slight to mild conductive or cochlear hearing loss. His HFT results, shown in Figure 4–6, were within normal limits (TPP = 40 daPa; magnitude compensated admittance = 0.25 mmho; component compensated admittance = 0.45 mmho).

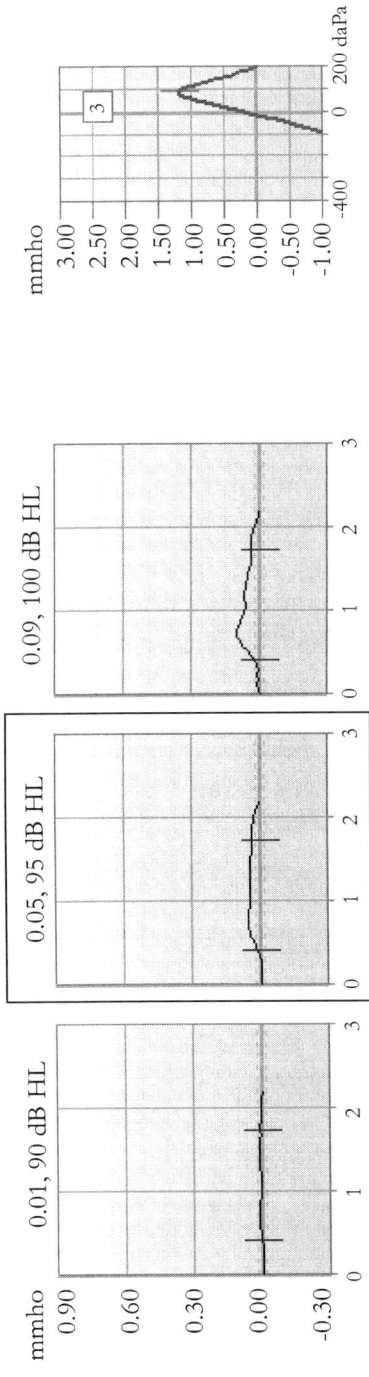

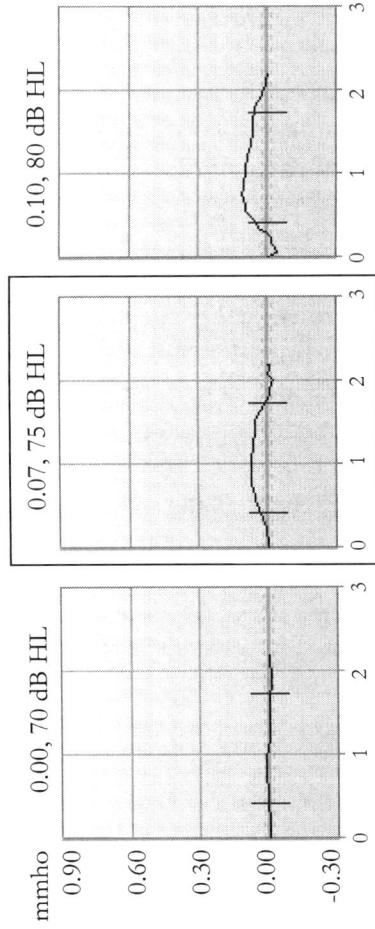

FIGURE 4–4. ASR findings obtained from a 2-day-old female (LT) who passed the AABR, HFT, and ASR tests, but failed the TEOAE test in her right ear. The results showed ASRTs of 95 and 75 dB HL at 0.5 and 4 kHz, respectively. The HFT results showed normal tympanometric findings with magnitude compensated admittance of 1.2 mmho at 90 daPa.

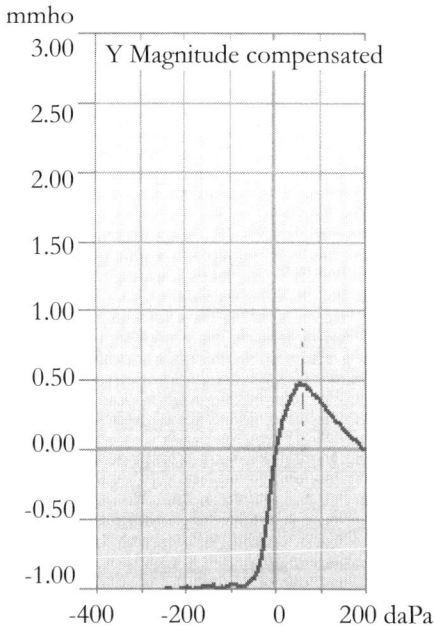

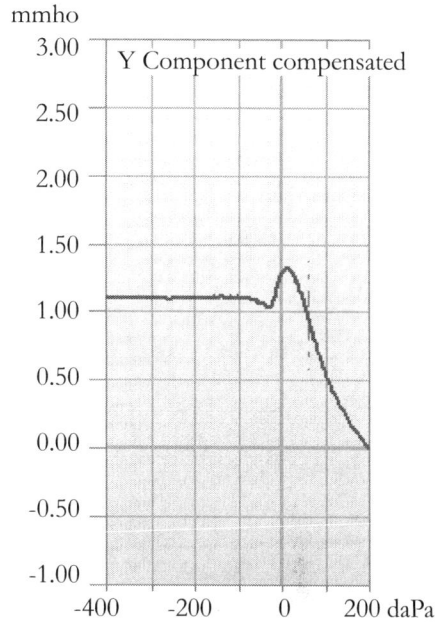

FIGURE 4–5. HFT findings obtained from a 2-day-old male (KS) who passed the AABR, HFT, and TEOAE tests, but failed the ASR test in his left ear. His HFT results indicate normal findings (TPP = 60 daPa; magnitude compensated admittance = 0.48 mmho; component compensated admittance = 1.3 mmho).

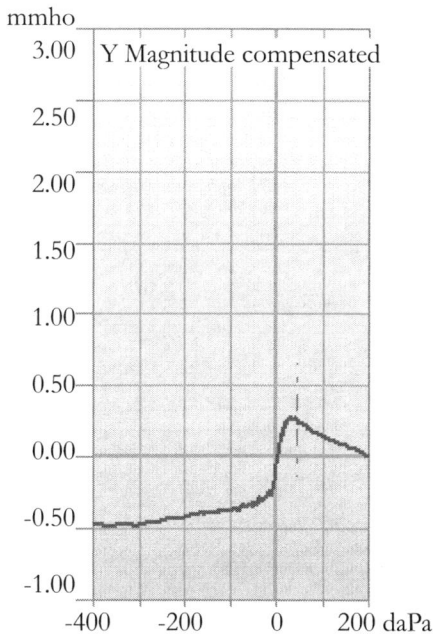

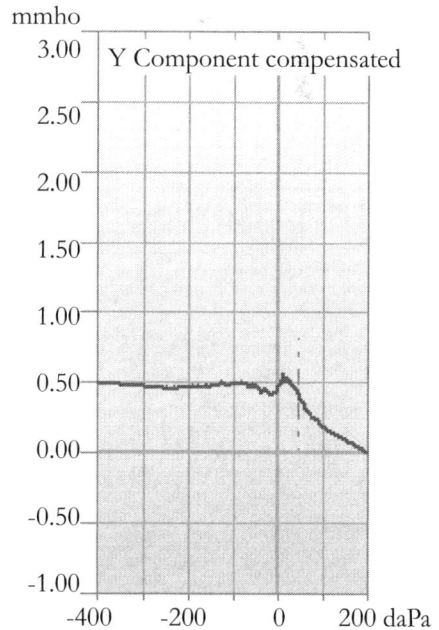

FIGURE 4–6. HFT findings obtained from a 2-day-old male (MJ) who passed the AABR and HFT, but failed the TEOAE and ASR tests in his right ear. The tympanograms showed a magnitude compensated admittance of 0.25 mmho and component compensated admittance of 0.45 mmho at 40 daPa.

81

Surprisingly, ipsilateral ASRs were absent. Hence, the absent ASRs, together with normal AABR, absent TEOAEs and normal HFT results suggest the possibility of a slight conductive loss. This conclusion is drawn based on the clinical experience that ASR is more sensitive to middle ear pathology than the HFT.

Case 6

Baby boy, RM, was born at 39 weeks of gestation with a birth weight of 2.7 kg.

He was 2 days old at the time of assessment. During the test, he was asleep. He passed the AABR screen and TEOAE test (SNR = −5, 6, 21, 20, and 24 dB at 1, 1.5, 2, 3, and 4 kHz, respectively) in the left ear. His HFT results, shown in Figure 4–7, indicate borderline normal findings (TPP = 30 daPa; magnitude compensated admittance = 0.2 mmho). Ipsilateral ASRs were present at normal levels (90, 70, 65, and 60 dB HL for the 0.5 kHz, 2 kHz, 4 kHz, and BBN, respectively). Although the borderline normal HFT results may raise a slight concern regarding the middle ear sta-

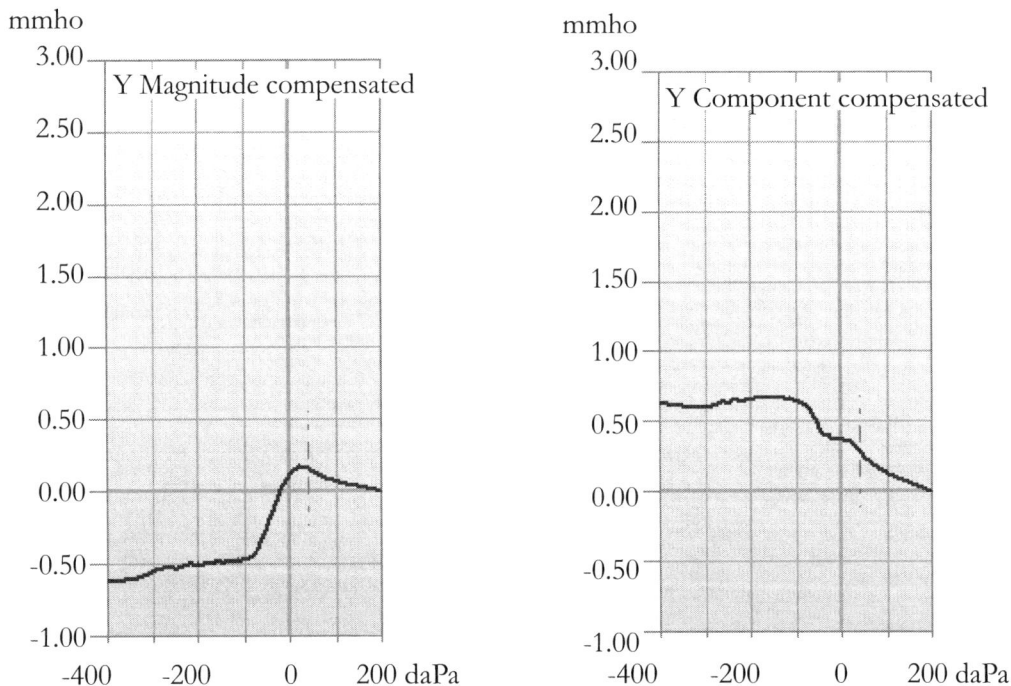

FIGURE 4–7. HFT findings obtained from a 2-day-old male (RM) who passed the AABR, TEOAE, and ASR tests in his left ear. His HFT results showed borderline normal findings with magnitude compensated admittance of 0.2 mmho at 30 daPa.

tus of RM's left ear, the normal AABR, TEOAE and ASR results suggest that RM should have normal auditory function up to the brainstem region.

Case 7

Baby girl, GS, was born at 40 weeks of gestation with a birth weight of 3.9 kg. She was 2 days old at the time of assessment. During the test, she was asleep. She passed the AABR screen and TEOAE

test in the left ear. Tympanometry findings indicate abnormal results with no positive peak as shown in Figure 4–8. Surprisingly, ipsilateral ASRs were present at normal levels (95, 75, 75, and 55 dB HL for the 0.5 kHz, 2 kHz, 4 kHz, and BBN, respectively). Taken together, the above results indicate grossly normal auditory function. The chance of middle ear dysfunction is slight because the presence of ASR at normal levels may exclude the possibility of significant middle ear pathology.

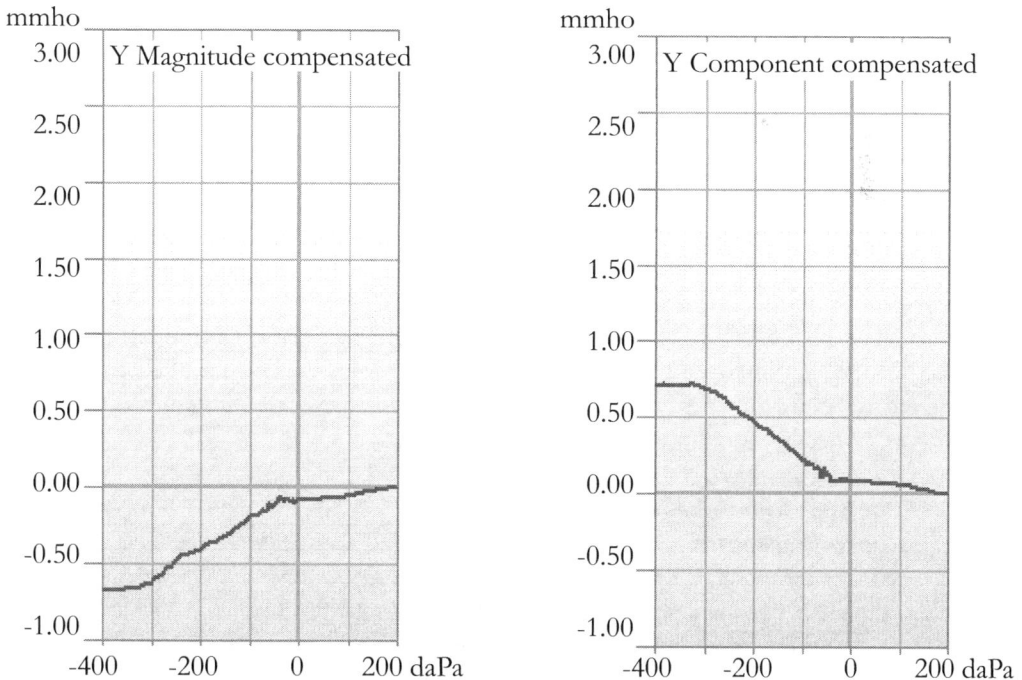

FIGURE 4–8. HFT findings obtained from a 2-day-old female (GS) who passed the AABR, TEOAE, and ASR tests in her left ear. Her HFT results indicate abnormal findings with no positive peak.

REFERENCES

Alford, B. R., Jerger, J., Coats, A. C., Peterson, P. R., & Weber, S. C. (1973). Neurophysiology of facial nerve testing. *Archives of Otolaryngology, 97*, 214–219.

Bennett, M. J., & Weatherby, L. A. (1979). Multiple probe frequency acoustic reflex measurements. *Scandinavian Audiology, 8*, 233–239.

Bennett, M. J., & Weatherby, L. A. (1982). Newborn acoustic reflexes to noise and puretone signals. *Journal of Speech and Hearing Research, 25*, 383–387.

Borg, E. (1968). A quantitative study of the effect of the acoustic stapedius reflex on sound transmission through the middle ear of man. *Acta Otolaryngologica* (Stockholm), *66*, 461–472.

Citron, D., & Adour, K. (1978). Acoustic reflex and loudness discomfort in acute facial paralysis. *Archives of Otolaryngology, 104*, 303–308.

Ferguson, M. A., Smith, P. A., Lutman, M. E., Mason, S. M., Coles, R. R. A., & Gibbin, K. B. (1996). Efficiency of tests used to screen cerebello-pontine angle tumors: A prospective study. *British Journal of Audiology, 30*, 159–176.

Geddes, N. (1987). Tympanometry and the stapedial reflex in the first five days of life. *International Journal of Pediatric Otorhinolaryngology, 13*, 293–297.

Gelfand, S.A. (1984). The contralateral acoustic reflex. In S. Silman (Ed.), *The acoustic reflex: Basic principles and clinical applications*. Orlando, FL: Academic Press.

Gelfand, S.A. (1994). Acoustic reflex threshold tenth percentiles and functional hearing impairment. *Journal of the American Academy of Audiology, 5*, 10–16.

Gelfand, S.A. (2009). The acoustic reflex. In J. Katz, L. Medwetsky, R. Burkard, & L. Hood. (Eds.), *Handbook of clinical audi-ology* (6th ed.). Baltimore, MD: Lippincott Williams & Wilkins.

Hall, J. W. (1978). Predicting hearing level from the acoustic reflex: A comparison of three methods. *Archives of Otolaryngology, 104*, 601–606.

Handler, S. D., & Margolis, R. H. (1977). Predicting hearing loss from stapedius reflex thresholds in patients with sensorineural impairment. *Annals of Otology, Rhinology and Laryngology, 84*, 425–431.

Hirsch, J. E., Margolis, R. H., & Rykken, J. R. (1992). A comparison of acoustic reflex and auditory brain stem response screening of high-risk infants. *Ear and Hearing, 13*, 181–186.

Holte, L., Margolis, R. H., & Cavanaugh, R. (1991). Developmental changes in multifrequency tympanograms. *Audiology, 30*, 1–24.

Jerger, J., Anthony, L., Jerger, S., & Mauldin, L. (1974a). Studies in impedance audiometry: III. Middle ear disorders. *Archives of Otolaryngology, 99*, 165–171.

Jerger, J., Burney, P., Mauldin, L., & Crump, B. (1974b). Predicting hearing loss from the acoustic reflex. *Journal of the Speech and Hearing Disorders, 39*, 11–17.

Jerger, J., Hayes, D., Anthony, L., & Mauldin, L. (1978). Factors influencing prediction of hearing levels from the acoustic reflex. *Monographs in Contemporary Audiology, 1*, 1–20.

Joint Committee on Infant Hearing (JCIH). (2007). Year 2007 Position Statement: Principles and guidelines for early detection and intervention programs. *Pediatrics, 120*, 898–921.

Kei, J. (in press). Acoustic stapedial reflexes in healthy neonates: Normative data and test-retest reliability. *Journal of the American Academy of Audiology.*

Keith, R. W., & Bench, R.J. (1978). Stapedial reflex in neonates. *Scandinavian Audiology, 7*, 187–191.

Marchant, C. D., McMillan, P. M., Shurin, P. A., Johnson, C. E., Turczyk, R. N., Feinstein, J. C., & Panek, D. M. (1986). Objective diagnosis of otitis media in early infancy by tympanometry and ipsilateral acoustic reflex thresholds. *Journal of Pediatrics, 109,* 590–595.

Mazlan, R., Kei, J., & Hickson, L. (2009). Test-retest reliability of acoustic reflex testing in healthy newborns. *Ear and Hearing, 30,* 295–301.

Mazlan, R., Kei, J., Hickson, L., Stapleton, C., Grant, S., Lim, S., . . . Linning, R. (2007). High frequency immittance findings: Newborn versus 6-week-old infants. *International Journal of Audiology, 46,* 711–717.

McMillan, P. M., Bennett, M. J., Marchant, C. D., & Shurin, P. A. (1985). Ipsilateral and contralateral acoustic reflexes in neonates. *Ear and Hearing, 6,* 320–324.

Moller, A. R. (1961). Bilateral contraction of the tympanic muscles in man. *Annals of Otology, Rhinology and Laryngology, 70,* 733–752.

Niemeyer, W., & Sesterhenn, G. (1974). Calculating the hearing threshold from the stapedius reflex threshold for different sound stimuli. *Audiology, 13,* 421–427.

Northern, J. L., & Downs, M. P. (2001). *Hearing in children* (5th ed.). Philadelphia, PA: Lippincott Williams & Wilkins.

Nozza, R., Bluestone, C. D., Kardatzke, D., & Bachman, R. (1992). Identification of middle ear effusion by aural acoustic admittance and otoscopy. *Ear and Hearing, 15,* 310–323.

Silman, S., & Silverman, C. A. (1991). *Audiology diagnosis: Principles and applications.* San Diego, CA: Academic Press.

Swanepoel, D. W., Werner, S., Hugo, R., Louw, B., Owen, R., & Swanepoel, A. (2007). High frequency immittance for neonates: A normative study. *Acta Otolaryngologica, 127,* 49–56.

Weatherby, L. A., & Bennett, M. J. (1980). The neonatal acoustic reflex. *Scandinavian Audiology, 9,* 103–110.

CHAPTER 5

Assessing Middle Ear Function in Humans Using Multifrequency Tympanometry: An Overview

FEI ZHAO AND JIE WANG

INTRODUCTION

Conventional tympanometry uses a single, low-frequency (usually 220 or 226 Hz) probe tone and measures the compliance of the middle ear system while the air pressure is varied in the external ear canal. It generally has been accepted as a routine procedure in otological assessment, which aims to detect different types of middle ear pathologies with associated changes in tympanometric patterns (Fowler & Shanks, 1997; Margolis & Hunter, 2002; Shanks, 1984). However, single-frequency tympanometry does not give a comprehensive

description of how sound of different frequencies is transmitted through the middle ear and to what extent sound is attenuated before it reaches the cochlea. Technologic advances in instrumentation have enabled the acoustical characteristics of the middle ear to be depicted using multifrequency tympanometry (MFT). MFT is a generic term to denote the measurement of middle ear characteristics using sound of more than one frequency. The MFT procedure may utilize a sweep frequency technique at multiple applied air pressures to the ear canal, a sweep pressure technique using sound of multiple discrete frequencies (Margolis & Goycoolea, 1993), or a wideband technique using a click or chirp at ambient pressure or applied pressure (Keefe, Ling, & Bulen, 1992). Several commercial MFT devices and research tools have been developed in recent years to provide important clinical information for identifying middle ear pathologies.

This chapter gives an overview on the current development of MFT and its clinical applications. By drawing together elements of the earlier chapters, this chapter aims to provide further insight into the middle ear dynamics in normal and pathologic middle ear systems, contributing to further clinical application of MFT and stimulate research in this fast developing area.

THE MIDDLE EAR

The middle ear is part of the peripheral auditory system. It is an air-filled cavity comprising of several structures as shown in Figure 5–1. The human middle ear consists of the tympanic membrane (TM), three ossicles (malleus, incus, and stapes), ligaments and tendons, and the bony middle ear cavity. There are two joints (incudomalleolar joint and incudostapedial joint) bridging the three ossicles and transferring sound energy into the perilymph of the inner ear. The human middle ear works as a mechanical system controlled by the middle ear mechanical components, that is, mass,

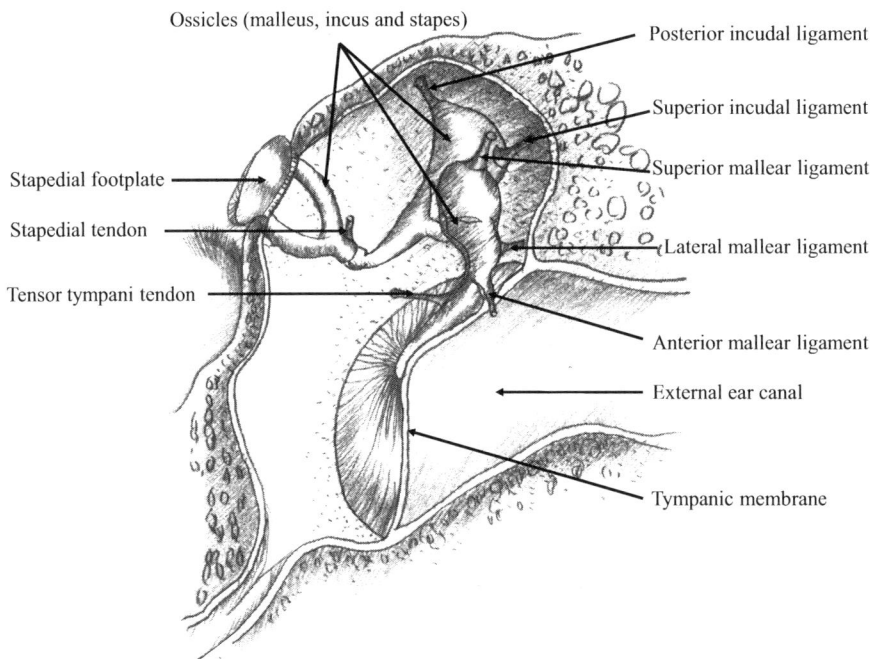

Ossicles (malleus, incus and stapes)
Posterior incudal ligament
Superior incudal ligament
Superior mallear ligament
Stapedial footplate
Stapedial tendon
Tensor tympani tendon
Lateral mallear ligament
Anterior mallear ligament
External ear canal
Tympanic membrane

FIGURE 5–1. Structure of the human middle ear.

stiffness, and friction, and plays an important role in sound transmission. Sound collected in the air-filled external ear is transformed into mechanical vibrations of the eardrum and ossicular chain, and then into a travelling wave in the fluid-filled cochlea in the inner ear.

The middle ear functions as an impedance-matching device between the low impedance of air and high impedance of cochlear fluids. This is achieved naturally by the mechanical structure of the middle ear, mainly due to the difference in the areas of the tympanic membrane and the stapes footplate and, to a lesser extent, the lever action of the ossicular chain (Figure 5–2) (Yost, 2000), that is, the effective TM vibration area is approximately 20 times greater than the area of the oval window, whereas the length of the malleus is 1.3 times longer than the long process of the incus. This increases the efficiency

with which sound energy is transferred from air to the fluid in the cochlea.

Middle ear mechanics can be altered as a result of the middle ear mechanical disturbances resulting from middle ear disorders, which can be detected by measuring the acoustic admittance of the middle ear system.

BASIC CONCEPTS— IMPEDANCE AND ADMITTANCE

In measuring middle ear function, the generic term acoustic immittance refers to acoustic impedance (Z_a) or acoustic admittance (Y_a). Figure 5–3 provides a summary of the relationship between acoustic impedance and admittance, together with their individual components. Both acoustic impedance and acoustic admittance are important concepts in

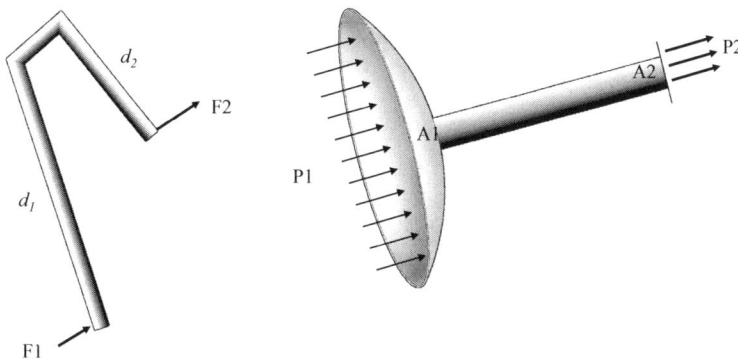

FIGURE 5–2. Mechanisms of sound pressure amplification by the middle ear system. (1) Lever action: a smaller force acts through a longer distance, resulting in a larger force acting through shorter distance; (2) Pressure amplification by piston action: a small pressure on a large area produces the same force as a large pressure on a small area.

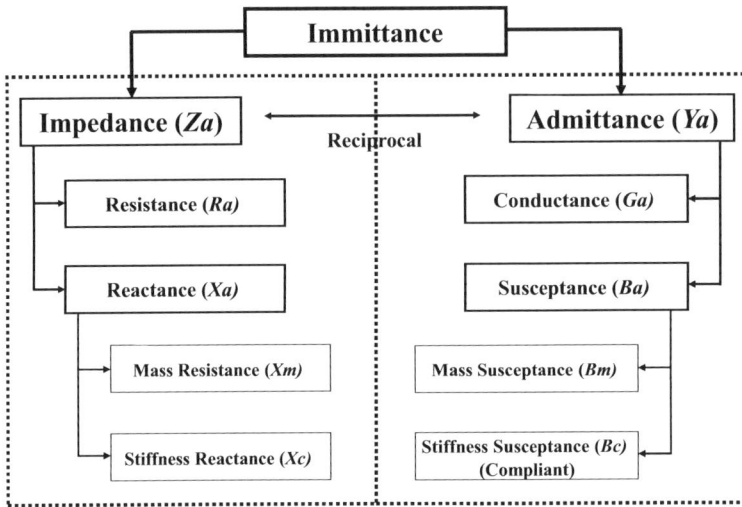

FIGURE 5–3. Immittance measures and their relationships.

terms of sound energy transmission in the middle ear system.

On the basis of the mathematic formula, the Z_a is the sum of the value of real part (R_a) and that of the imaginary part (X_a, i denotes the imaginary number), that is,

$$Z_a = R_a + iX_a \qquad \text{Eqn. (1)}$$

or

$$Z_a = \sqrt{R_a^2 + X_a^2} \qquad \text{Eqn. (2)}$$

where R_a and X_a represent acoustic resistance and acoustic reactance, respectively.

The middle ear system is analogous to a mechanical system consisting of a mass, spring and friction. In Equation (1), Z_a comprises three components: mass, stiffness, and resistance. The mass component includes the tympanic membrane, ossicles, and air in the external

acoustic canal and middle ear cavity. The stiffness component consists of the tympanic membrane, the joint of incudo-stapedial and incudomalleal, the ligaments/tendons (Shanks, 1984). The X_a in Equation (1) consists of the compliant reactance (X_c) associated with the spring and mass reactance (X_m) associated with the mass. X_c and X_m act against each other. The acoustic resistance (R_a) represents the frictional component, which impedes the flow of sound through the vibratory middle ear system (Shanks, 1984).

From the relationship shown in Figure 5–3, the acoustic admittance (Y_a) is the reciprocal of acoustic impedance (Z_a), that is,

$$Y_a = 1/Z_a \qquad \text{Eqn. (3)}$$

Similar to the acoustic impedance (Z_a), Y_a is the sum of the real part of conductance G_a and imaginary part of susceptance B_a as show in the following equations:

$$Y_a = G_a + iB_a \qquad \text{Eqn. (4)}$$

or

$$Y_a = \sqrt{G_a^2 + B_a^2} \qquad \text{Eqn. (5)}$$

where G_a and B_a represent acoustic conductance and acoustic susceptance, respectively.

Similar to the acoustic impedance, the acoustic admittance (Y_a) is made up of three components: mass susceptance (B_M, inverse of X_m), compliant susceptance (B_C, inverse of X_c) and conductance (G_a, inverse of R_a). On the basis of equations mentioned above, the two directional quantities Z_a and Y_a can be represented as shown in Figure 5–4. In addition, Z_a and Y_a vary systematically as a function of frequency of sound because both the susceptance and reactance components are frequency dependent.

EFFECT OF PROBE-TONE FREQUENCY ON ADMITTANCE

The relationship between the admittance components and probe frequencies has been widely investigated (Colletti, 1975, 1976; Holte, Margolis, & Cavanaugh, 1991; Kei et al., 2003; Shahnaz & Polka, 2002). In general, as the frequency increases, the total susceptance value progresses from positive (indicating a stiffness-controlled middle ear system) to zero (indicating resonance of the middle ear), and then negative (indicating a mass-controlled middle ear system). Consequently, different tympanometric configurations can be observed depending on the probe frequencies.

Vanhuyse, Creten, and Van Camp (1975) described in detail the effect of probe frequency on tympanometric configurations. In establishing their mathematical model, reactance (R) was assumed to be monotonically decreasing

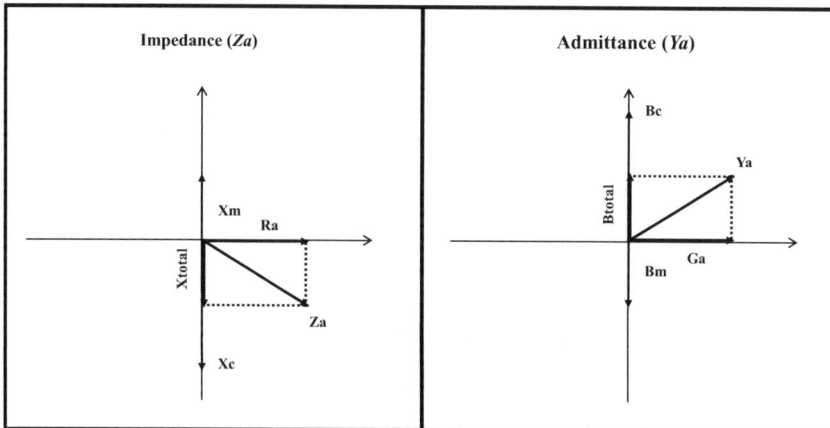

FIGURE 5–4. Acoustic impedance (Z_a) and acoustic admittance (Y_a) represented by rectangular coordinates.

as a function of increasing air pressure in the ear canal, with a higher resistance at the negative pressure than that at the positive pressure end. As the reactance increases from negative to positive values with increasing probe frequencies, four different tympanometric patterns were found. Each pattern was classified according to the number of notches in the susceptance (B) and conductance (G) tympanograms. The four patterns are 1B1G, 3B1G, 3B3G, and 5B3G, as described in Table 5–1. Despite the complex interaction between tympanogram and probe frequency, the configuration of the susceptance and conductance tympanograms can be predicted using the Vanhuyse model. The tympanometric patterns provide useful information for evaluating the function of the middle ear.

TABLE 5–1. Four Tympanometric Patterns Using the Vanhuyse Model and Interpretations

Pattern in the Vanhuyse Model	Brief Description and Interpretation
1B1G B G	One susceptance peak and one conductance peak. It occurs when the susceptance is greater than the conductance. This 1B1G tympanogram indicates a stiffness-dominated middle ear system.
3B1G B G	Three susceptance notches and one conductance peak. This 3B1G pattern indicates that the middle ear is less dominated by the stiffness. With the stiffness of the middle ear decreasing to zero, the middle ear begins to be dominated by mass, and the probe frequency is equal to the resonance frequency of the middle ear. This is an important stage of transition from a stiffness-controlled to mass-controlled middle ear system.
3B3G B G	Three susceptance and three conductance notches. This 3B3G pattern occurs when the middle ear is primarily mass controlled, showing the susceptance values being negative, but smaller than the conductance at the low pressure and greater in absolute value than conductance at high pressures.
5B3G B G	This 5B3G pattern occurs when the mass susceptance increases and becomes larger in magnitude than the conductance.

DEVELOPMENT OF MULTIPLE FREQUENCY TYMPANOMETRY (MFT)

Tympanometry is a procedure used in the assessment of middle ear function, in which the immittance of the tympanic membrane and middle ear is measured as a function of ear canal air pressure. Conventional tympanometry with a single low-frequency probe tone (220 or 226 Hz) is routinely used in audiology clinics as part of the audiologic assessment battery. In contrast, the MFT measures middle ear function by using multiple probe tone frequencies. Both components of admittance (susceptance and conductance) are measured either at an individual frequency or across a wide frequency range (e.g., from 200 to 2000 Hz). Essentially, MFT provides a more comprehensive view of the function of the middle ear than single-frequency tympanometry.

Early Research in MFT

Pioneer research of MFT was carried out by Professor Vittorio Colletti in the 1970s (Colletti, 1975, 1976, 1977). In these studies, tympanograms were recorded from normal and pathologic ears using the probe tone frequencies ranging from 0.2 to 2.0 kHz. Distinguishable probe frequency regions associated with typical tympanometric patterns were found in both normal and abnormal middle ears as the probe frequency was increased. For example, Colletti (1977) showed that a "W" tympanometric pattern occurred at the frequency region around 900 to 1000 Hz in normal middle ears. But the "W" tympanometric pattern also occurred in patients with ossicular discontinuity only when the probe frequency was decreased to between 500 and 900 Hz. Hence, the probe frequency at which the "W" tympanometric pattern occurs appears to be a good indicator for distinguishing normal from certain pathological middle ears (Shahnaz & Polka, 1997). The mechanism behind this is likely due to the reduction in the mass component of the middle ear transmission system, which subsequently decreases the middle-ear resonance frequency. In addition, in the ears with stapes fixation, the "W" tympanometric pattern occurred at the frequency region between 850 and 1650 Hz, which was consistent with an increase in stiffness and a concomitant increase in the middle-ear resonance frequency. However, as indicated above, the range of probe frequencies showing the "W" tympanometric pattern in patients with stapedial fixation or ossicular discontinuity overlapped to a certain extent with that for normal middle ears (Miani, Bergamin, Barotti, & Isola, 2000).

Modern MFT Devices and Their Features

Devices for measuring middle ear function have evolved from a mechanical acoustic bridge to electroacoustic bridge, and then to computer-based tympanometers. After more than 30 years since the

MFT was first developed, contemporary tympanometers are capable of versatile and sophisticated clinical measurements with the help of the digital signal processing (DSP) technology. Currently, there are several commercially available MFT devices, such as the GSI Tymstar (or GSI 33 version 2), Madsen Otoflex 100, and Kamplex Impedance Audiometer. Table 5–2 shows five tympanometers with various advanced features.

As seen in Table 5–2, most devices have the facility to choose the type of immittance measures, display of the tympanogram and paradigms for data acquisition. For example, the MFT device can be connected to a computer with custom-made software to select different test options and protocols. Furthermore, the computer-driven device enables convenient data collection, storage, analysis, and report. The Madsen Otoflex 100 utilizes Bluetooth technology to enable the device to move around easily when testing young patients, thus improving its flexibility.

Emerging MFT Instruments

Apart from those commercial devices mentioned previously, new MFT instruments are being developed, which utilize a wider frequency range of measurements. They are sweep frequency impedance (SFI) meter and wideband energy reflectance (WBER, also previously called Otoreflectance, and currently commercialized as Wideband Tympanometry [WBT]) (e.g., Keefe et al., 1992; Margolis, Saly, & Keefe, 1999;

Wada, Koike, & Kobayashi, 1998). The SFI was developed by Professor Hiroshi Wada and his colleagues in 1989 to record sound pressure in the ear canal in dB SPL across a sweeping stimulus frequency (Wada, Kobayashi, Suetake, & Tachizaki, 1989). The SFI test has advantages over the traditional admittance measures by providing dynamic characteristics of the middle ear represented in two- and three-dimensional graphs. These characteristics include measures of resonance frequency and mobility of the middle ear system (Wada et al., 1998; Zhao, Wada, Koike, Ohyama, Kawase, & Stephens, 2002, 2003).

The other MFT device, the WBER, is designed to assess wideband acoustic transfer functions (ATFs) of the middle ear. A loudspeaker delivers a sound (click or chirp) to the ear. Although some of the sound energy is transmitted into the middle ear, a proportion of it is reflected back from the TM. A microphone measures this reflected response along with the incident signal from the loudspeaker. By comparing sound pressure between the reflected and incident signal at various frequencies, the transmission characteristics of sound through the middle ear can be depicted. To date, a few studies have suggested that the WBER can differentiate normal from abnormal middle ears (Feeney, Grant, & Marryott, 2003; Keefe et al., 1992; Margolis et al., 1999; Shahnaz, Bork, Polka, Longridge, Bell, & Westerberg, 2009; Zhao, Lowe, Meredith, & Rhodes, 2008; Zhao, Meredith, Wotherspoon, & Rhodes, 2007).

Overall, both SFI and WBER have shown great potential to be used in

TABLE 5–2. Five Multiple/High-Frequency Tympanometry Devices for Measuring Middle Ear Function

Equipment	Probe Frequency (Hz)	General Features	Specific Features
Virtual Model 310	226, 633/678,1000	• Low frequency tympanometry • Acoustic reflex threshold test • Acoustic tone decay test • Eustachian tube function (ETF) test	• Sweep frequency measurement • Two components tympanometry • Admittance-phase angle measurement
GSI 33 (Ver. 2) or TympStar2	226-1000	• Low frequency tympanometry • Acoustic reflex threshold test • Acoustic tone decay test • ETF test	• Sweep frequency measurement • Two components tympanometry • PC interface
GN Otometrics—Madsen Otoflex 100	226, 1000	• Low frequency tympanometry • Acoustic reflex threshold test • Acoustic tone decay test • ETF test	• Comprehensive PC interface • Two-component tympanometry • Bluetooth technology • Measurements done in OTO-suite can be transferred to other systems using Extensible Markup Language (XML) data format
GN Otometrics—Madsen Capella,	226, 1000	• Screening tympanometry	• Software-based modular • Combined with OAE system
Kamplex (KLT25) Impedance Audiometer	226, 678, 800, 1000	• Low frequency tympanometry • Acoustic reflex threshold test • Acoustic tone decay test • ETF test	• Combined with audiometry modular • PC interface

adults and young infants by providing more information about the dynamical behavior of the middle ear (Beers, Shahnaz, Westerberg, & Kozak, 2010; Keefe, Folsom, Gorga, Vohr, Bulen, & Norton, 2000; Keefe, Gorga, Neely, Zhao, & Vohr, 2003; Keefe, Zhao, Neely, Gorga, & Vohr, 2003; Merchant, Horton, & Voss, 2010; Shahnaz, Miranda, & Polka, 2008; Vander Werff, Prieve, & Georgantas, 2007). It is not only these functional reasons that make them attractive tools, the measures are also simple, fast, objective, reproducible and noninvasive. Furthermore, plotting a three-dimensional graph by frequency as a function of ear-canal pressure has been developed as an additional feature to these MFTs. Such a three-dimensional approach by recording detailed complex components provides virtual visual images for better understanding of important dynamic characteristics in the middle ear transmission system. The detailed mechanisms and their clinical applications are discussed in Chapters 6 and 7.

CHARACTERISTICS OF MFT AND ITS APPLICATION

Characteristics of MFT in Subjects with Normal Middle Ear Function

Normative data obtained from MFT are essential for separating normal middle ears from ears with middle ear pathology. As described in the previous section, the tympanometric pattern obtained from a normal middle ear progresses through a systematic sequence from 1B1G to 5B3G when the probe frequency increases. The 1B1G pattern was primarily recorded in normal adult ears using low-frequency probe tones and in approximately 75% of normal adult ears using probe tones of 660/678 Hz (Vanhuyse et al., 1975). In contrast, the 3B1G pattern primarily occurred in normal adult ears when a high-frequency probe tone such as 1 kHz was used. However, this 3B1G pattern was also recorded in approximately 20% of normal adults when the probe frequency was lower than 660/678 Hz (Margolis, Van Camp, Wilson, & Creten, 1985). With the use of high probe tone frequencies, only 8% and 5% of normal middle ears showed the 3B3G and 5B3G patterns, respectively.

Another important characteristic feature of MFT is associated with the measurement of resonance frequency of the middle ear. As discussed previously, the contributions of compliant susceptance and mass susceptance vary as a function of probe frequency. Although the compliant susceptance component dominates at low frequencies, the mass susceptance dominates at high frequencies. At a certain frequency when the compliant susceptance and mass susceptance are equal and opposite in direction, the effect of the mass and spring elements of the middle ear cancel each other. When this happens, the middle ear is said to be in resonance. The frequency at which resonance occurs is called the resonance frequency (RF) of the middle ear.

Table 5–3 shows a summary of findings from nine studies which measured RF using various commercial and custom-made devices. These studies showed that the RF of a normal middle ear falls between 560 and 2000 Hz (e.g., Hanks & Mortensen, 1997; Shahnaz & Polka, 1997; Shanks, Wilson, & Cambron, 1993; Valvik, Johnsen, & Laukli, 1994; Wada et al., 1998). Such a wide normative range of resonance frequency is likely associated with various influencing factors, such as demographic variations, different instruments and measuring techniques (Margolis & Goycoolea, 1993; Margolis & Smith, 1977; Shahnaz & Davies, 2006; Shanks et al., 1993).

In general, the measurement of RF provides potential diagnostic value in that mass loading pathologies (such as ossicular discontinuity) are known to be associated with decreased stiffness and a lowering of RF, whereas pathologies that increase middle ear stiffness (such as otosclerosis) have been shown to increase the RF (Colletti, 1975, 1976, 1977; Lilly, 1973; Van Camp & Vogeleer, 1986; Zwislocki, 1982). However, the normal range of the resonance frequency is quite wide, even though confounding variables were properly controlled in these studies (as shown in Table 5–3). Therefore, interpretation of RF results should be made cautiously, and necessarily in combination with other information obtained from MFT. In addition, clinical information other than tympanometric assessment results such as case history, otoscopy and audiometric results may help with the diagnosis of middle ear disorders.

Clinical Application of MFT in Adult Patients with Middle Ear Disorders

In ears with pathological conditions of the middle ear, the mechanics of the middle ear system is disturbed, resulting in inefficient transmission of sound energy through the middle ear and a shift of RF of the middle ear. Although substantial evidence has shown that conventional low-frequency tympanometry can detect many middle ear disorders, it has proved to be relatively insensitive to some middle ear pathological conditions. To improve the accuracy of diagnosis of these conditions, researchers have explored the use of MFT as an alternative measure. For example, tympanic membrane aberrations such as minor scarring, retracted tympanic membrane and tympanosclerosis are not readily detected by conventional low-frequency tympanometry (Maw & Bawden, 1994). Interestingly, MFT findings reveal a significant higher RF of the middle ear in patients with high-stiffness tympanic membrane abnormalities, such as retracted tympanic membrane and tympanosclerosis, than that in people with normal middle ear function (Valvik et al., 1994). In contrast, the RF for low-stiffness tympanometric conditions, such as tympanic membrane atrophy, is lower when compared to that for normal middle ear conditions (Hunter & Margolis, 1997).

Otitis media with effusion (OME) is the most common cause for hearing loss in children. In most studies of OME, ears showed either a type B or type C

TABLE 5–3. Summary of Findings from Studies on Measuring Resonance Frequency in Individuals with Normal Middle Ear Function Using MFT Devices

Authors	Equipment and Measurement	Subjects	Resonance Frequency (RF) Criteria and Normal Range
Hanks & Rose (1993)	*GSI 33 (Ver. 2)* 1. A frequency sweep increment of 50 Hz from 250 to 2000 Hz. 2. Tympanogram at a pressure range of −400 to +200 daPa, starting from +200 daPa.	158 children (aged 12–15 yr); 68 with severe to profound SNHL and 90 with normal hearing.	Criteria: Compensated susceptance (positive tail) = 0 RF (+200) = 1003 ± 216 Hz (90% range: 650–1400 Hz)
Valvik et al. (1994)	*GSI 33 (Ver. 2)* 1. Tympanogram was measured at 200 daPa (Y_{+200}); 2. Admittance at a pressure corresponding to the peak of the conventional tympanogram (Y_{peak}) 3. Difference between Y_{+200} and Y_{peak} was calculated as a function of frequency.	100 ears with normal middle ear function.	Criteria: Compensated susceptance (positive tail) = 0 RF (+200) = 1049 ± 261Hz
Hanks & Mortensen (1997)	*GSI 33 (Ver. 2)* 1. A frequency sweep increment of 50 Hz from 250 to 2000 Hz. 2. Tympanogram at a pressure range of −400 to +200 daPa, starting from +200 daPa. 3. Tympanogram at a pressure range of +200 to −400 daPa, starting from −400 daPa.	106 ears of 53 subjects (25 males; 28 females) with normal hearing and middle ear function. Age = 18–25 yr.	Criteria: Compensated susceptance (positive tail or negative tail) = 0 RF (+200) = 908 ± 188 (90% range: 650–1300 Hz) RF (−400) = 1318 ± 308 (90% range: 900–1750 Hz)

continues

Authors	Equipment and Measurement	Subjects	Resonance Frequency (RF) Criteria and Normal Range
Shanks, Wilson, & Cambron (1993)	*Virtual 310* 1. Susceptance and conductance tympanograms were recorded using 10 probe tone frequencies between 226 and 1243 Hz (113 Hz intervals); 2. Tympanogram at a pressure range of −350 to +200 daPa;	26 male subjects with normal hearing and middle ear function (aged 20–40 yr, mean age = 29.7 yr).	Criteria: Compensated susceptance (positive tail or negative tail) = 0 RF (+200) = 817 Hz (90% range: 565–1130 Hz) RF (−350) = 1100 Hz (90% range: 678–1234 Hz)
Margolis & Goycoolea (1993)	*Virtual 310* 1. "Sweep frequency method": Susceptance and conductance tympanograms were recorded using 20 probe-tone frequencies between 250 and 2000 Hz (1/6 octave step intervals) at a fixed ear canal air pressure, ranging from +400 to −500 daPa in 14 daPa steps. 2. "Sweep pressure method": Probe frequency was fixed as the air pressure was swept from +400 to −500 at a rate of 250 daPa/sec.	56 ears of 28 normal hearing subjects (14 males; 14 females); Age = 19–48 yr.	Criteria: Compensated susceptance (positive tail or negative tail or two tails) = 0 *Sweep frequency method:* RF (+200) = 1135 ± 306 Hz (90% range: 800–2000 Hz) RF (−500) = 1315 ± 377 Hz (90% range: 710–2000 Hz) RF (2tails) = 1223 ± 332 Hz (90% range: 630–1400 Hz) *Sweep pressure method:* RF (+200) = 990 ± 290 Hz (90% range: 800–2000 Hz) RF (−500) = 1132 ± 337 Hz (90% range: 710–2000 Hz) RF (2tails) = 1063 ± 313 Hz (90% range: 630–2000 Hz)

TABLE 5–3. *continued*

Authors	Equipment and Measurement	Subjects	Resonance Frequency (RF) Criteria and Normal Range
Holte (1996)	*Virtual 310* Sweeping frequency from 250 through 2000 Hz (while holding air pressure in the ear canal constant at intervals of 20 daPa from +250 to –300 daPa)	144 male subjects with normal hearing and middle ear function. 20 subjects in each decade of life from 20 to 79 yr of age; 16 subjects older than 79 yr, including three older than 90 yr.	Criteria: Compensated susceptance (positive tail or negative tail) = 0 RF (+250) = 906 ± 184 Hz (90% range: 630–1250 Hz) RF (–300) = 1001 ± 257 (90% range: 710–1400 Hz)
Shahnaz & Polka (1997)	*Virtual 310* 1. "Sweep frequency method": Susceptance and conductance tympanograms were recorded using 20 probe tone frequencies between 250 and 2000 Hz (1/6 octave step intervals) at a fixed ear canal air pressure, ranging from +250 to –300 daPa in 9 daPa steps. 2. "Sweep pressure method": Probe frequency was fixed as the air pressure was swept from +250 to –300 at a rate of 125 daPa/sec.	36 subjects (68 ears) with normal hearing and middle ear function (mean age = 22 yr; range = 20–43 yr).	Criteria: Compensated susceptance (positive tail or negative tail) = 0 *Sweep frequency method:* RF (+250) = 894 ± 166 Hz (90% range: 630–1120 Hz) RF (–300) = 1043 ± 290 Hz (90% range: 710–1400 Hz) *Sweep pressure method:* RF (+250) = 789 ± 53 Hz (90% range: 560–1000 Hz) RF (–300) = 924 ± 240 Hz (90% range: 865–982 Hz)

Authors	Equipment and Measurement	Subjects	Resonance Frequency (RF) Criteria and Normal Range
Wada et al. (1998)	*Sweep frequency impedance (SFI) meter* 1. The SFI records sound pressure in the ear canal in dB SPL across a sweeping stimulus frequency from 0.1 to 2.0 kHz 2. The static pressure of the external ear canal is varied between −300 and +200 daPa at 50 daPa intervals.	275 ears with intact tympanic membrane and normal hearing function	Criteria: midpoint of the frequencies corresponding to variation between the maximum and minimum sound pressures. RF = 1170 ± 270 Hz
Wiley et al. (1999)	*Virtual 310* 1. Sweeping frequency from 250 through 2000 Hz; 2. Tympanometric measures were collected over a pressure range from +250 to −300 using a positive to negative direction at a rate of 100 daPa/sec.	404 subjects with normal hearing and middle ear function (aged 19–48 yrs).	Criteria: Compensated susceptance (positive tail or negative tail) = 0 RF (+250) = 866 ± 175 Hz RF (−300) = 1039 ± 283Hz

tympanogram using conventional low-frequency tympanometry. It has been suggested that MFT can provide more detailed information about middle ear dynamic characteristics in patients with OME. For example, Kontrogianni, Ferekidis, Ntouniadakis, Psarommatis, Apostolopoulos, and Adamopoulos (1996) found statistically significant decreases in both RF values and changes in phase angle in ears with OME when compared to normative data. These results are attributed to a mass-dominated middle ear mechanism caused by fluid in the middle ear.

Otosclerosis is an inherited disorder of bone growth that mainly affects the stapes and the bony labyrinth of the cochlea. The disorder is characterized by resorption of the normally hard bone and its replacement with newer, softer bone tissue that is highly spongy and vascularized. This spongy bone growth can eventually turn into a dense sclerotic mass (Newby & Popelka, 1992). These pathological changes impede the vibration of the stapes, resulting in a progressive conductive hearing loss at the initial stages of the disorder. As mentioned previously, low-frequency tympanometry is fairly sensitive to ossicular pathology because the tympanogram obtained reflects mainly stiffness-controlled components with little information on mass-controlled components such as the ossicular chain. Jerger, Anthony, Jerger, and Maudlin (1974) found that 95% of patients with otosclerosis had type A tympanogram using low-frequency tympanometry. Moreover, Muchink, Hildesheimer, Rubinstein, and Glettman (1989),

using both 220 Hz and 660 Hz probe tones, found that only one-third of the otosclerotic ears had low admittance values, whereas the remaining two-thirds showed admittance values in the normal or high ranges. In summary, the results from the above two studies showed a significant overlap of tympanometric results between normal and otosclerotic ears, which severely limits the diagnostic utility of low frequency tympanometry for identification of otosclerosis.

Using MFT with frequency of tone sweeping from 0.22 to 2.0 kHz, Colletti, Fiorino, Sittoni, and Policante (1993) measured RFs in normal subjects, otosclerotic patients and subjects who had undergone stapes surgery. They found that the otosclerotic group had high RFs, whereas stapedectomized subjects had low RF, when compared to normative RF data. Valvik et al. (1994) also found that patients with otosclerosis showed significantly higher RF than their normally hearing counterparts. Moreover, Shahnaz and Polka (2002) succeeded in distinguishing healthy from otosclerotic ears by measuring the admittance phase angle of 45° of the middle ear system using a probe tone of 630 Hz.

To date, the MFT has also been used to identify patients with ossicular chain separation (OCS) caused by trauma, sepsis or congenital abnormality. Although the low-frequency tympanometry shows abnormally high static admittance in cases with OCS, various studies have proved that the MFT demonstrates its advantages over low-frequency tympanometry by providing more information of this mass-related middle ear pathology. For example, the "W" typmanometric pattern and resonance frequency measured in patients with OCS have distinguishable diagnostic value, indicating an increase in the mass or a decrease in the stiffness of the middle ear transmission system (Colletti, 1977; Van Camp, Margolis, Wilson, Creten, & Shanks, 1986).

MAIN BENEFITS AND BARRIERS OF APPLYING MFT IN AUDIOLOGY/ENT CLINICS

When compared with low-frequency tympanometry, the overall benefits of applying MFT in Audiology/ENT clinics are: (1) improved validity for examining the middle ear status in infants and neonates; (2) improved sensitivity and specificity for testing ossicular pathological conditions; (3) provision of additional clinical information when borderline results are obtained from low-frequency tympanometry; and (4) provision of dynamic characteristics of the middle ear for ascertaining the resonance frequency and mobility of the middle ear.

Despite the above benefits, there are barriers that may hinder the widespread use of MFT in Audiology/ENT clinics. The main issues are: (1) MFT appears more complex with regard to the test procedure and interpretation of results; (2) the calibration of tympanometric instruments relies on the assumption that the ear canal behaves as a pure acoustic compliance. Because this assumption is not valid above 2000

Hz, it would be difficult to calibrate the probe sounds. Consequently, MFT cannot be performed correctly above 2000 Hz using conventional calibration methods; and (3) there are limited normative data and inadequate guidance for identifying middle ear pathological conditions in infants and adults.

CONCLUSION AND FUTURE RESEARCH

Although low frequency tympanometry has proved useful in diagnosing many common middle ear pathologies due to its ease of use and easy interpretation, it lacks the sensitivity to detect certain middle ear pathologies. On the contrary, MFT has been found to be sensitive to pathologies associated with ossicular chain abnormality. With continuing research, the MFT will be a promising diagnostic tool that serves as an alternative/additional test for the evaluation of middle ear pathologies.

In future research, standardizing the MFT procedures and optimizing methods of data analysis will be necessary. In particular, more MFT data are needed from large number of subgroups of patients with well-defined middle ear pathologies (e.g., serous otitis media, acute otitis media with effusion, tympanic membrane perforation, otosclerosis, cholesteatoma, discontinuity of the ossicular chain) to determine the sensitivity and specificity of the MFT. Furthermore, information on the relationship between MFT findings and other audiometric findings could make an important contribution to the clinical application of MFT. Finally, predicting MFT results using a computational model of the middle ear may be possible. This model will be useful for understanding the dynamic behavior of normal ears and ears with middle ear disorders.

REFERENCES

Beers, A. N., Shahnaz, N., Westerberg, B. D., & Kozak, F. K (2010). Wideband reflectance in normal Caucasian and Chinese school-aged children and in children with otitis media with effusion. *Ear and Hearing*, *31*, 221–233.

Colletti, V. (1975). Methodologic observations on tympanometry with regard to the probe tone frequency. *Acta Otolaryngologica*, *80*, 54–60.

Colletti, V. (1976). Tympanometry from 200 to 2000 Hz probe tone. *Audiology*, *15*, 106–119.

Colletti, V. (1977). Multifrequency tympanometry. *Audiology*, *16*, 278–287.

Colletti, V., Fiorino, F., Sittoni, V., & Policante, Z. (1993). Mechanics of the middle ear in otosclerosis and stapedoplasty. *Acta Otolaryngologica (Stockholm)*, *113*, 637–641.

Feeney, M. P., Grant, I. L., & Marryott, L. P. (2003). Wideband energy reflectance measurements in adults with middle-ear disorders. *Journal of Speech, Language, and Hearing Research*, *46*, 901–911.

Fowler, C. G., & Shanks, J. E. (1997). Tympanometry. In J. Katz, L. Medwetsky, R. Burkard, & L. Hood (Eds.), *Handbook of clinical audiology* (6th ed.). Baltimore, MD: Lippincott Williams & Wilkins.

Hanks, W. D., & Mortensen, B. A. (1997). Multifrequency tympanometry: Effects of ear canal volume compensation on middle ear resonance. *Journal of the American Academy of Audiology*, *8*, 53–58.

Hanks, W. D., & Rose, K. J. (1993). Middle ear resonance and acoustic immittance measures in children. *Journal of Speech and Hearing Research*, *36*, 218–222.

Holte, L. (1996). Aging effects in multifrequency tympanometry. *Ear and Hearing*, *17*, 12–18.

Holte, L. A., Margolis, R. H., & Cavanaugh, R. M. (1991). Developmental changes in multifrequency tympanograms. *Audiology*, *30*, 1–24.

Hunter, L. L., & Margolis, R. H. (1997). Effects of tympanic membrane abnormalities on auditory function. *Journal of the American Academy of Audiology*, *8*, 431–446.

Jerger, J., Anthony, L., Jerger, S., & Maudlin, L. (1974). Studies in impedance audiometry: III. Middle ear disorders. *Archives of Otolaryngology*, *99*, 165–171.

Keefe, D. H., Folsom, R., Gorga, M. P., Vohr, B. R., Bulen, J. C., & Norton, S. (2000). Identification of neonatal hearing impairment: Ear-canal measurements of acoustic admittance and reflectance in neonates. *Ear and Hearing*, *21*, 443–461.

Keefe, D. H., Gorga, M. P., Neely, S. T., Zhao, F., & Vohr, B. R. (2003). Ear-canal acoustic admittance and reflectance measurements in human neonates. II. Predictions of middle-ear in dysfunction and sensorineural hearing loss. *Journal of the Acoustical Society of America*, *113*, 407–422.

Keefe, D. H., Ling, R., & Bulen, J. C. (1992). Method to measure acoustic impedance and reflection coefficient. *Journal of the Acoustical Society of America*, *91*, 470–485.

Keefe, D. H., Zhao, F., Neely, S. T., Gorga, M. P., & Vohr, B. R. (2003). Ear-canal acoustic admittance and reflectance effects in human neonates. I. Predictions of otoacoustic emission and auditory brainstem responses. *Journal of the Acoustical Society of America*, *113*, 389–406.

Kei, J., Allison-Levrick, J., Dockray, J., Harrys, R., Kirkegard, C., Wong, J., . . . Tudehope, D. (2003). High frequency (1000 Hz) tympanometry in normal neonates. *Journal of the American Academy of Audiology, 14,* 20–28.

Kontrogianni, A., Ferekidis, E., Ntouniadakis, E., Psarommatis, I., Apostolopoulos, N., & Adamopoulos, G. (1996). Multiple-frequency tympanometry in children with otitis media with effusion. *Journal for Oto-Rhino-Laryngology-Head and Neck Surgery, 58,* 78–81.

Lilly, D. (1973). Measurement of acoustic impedance at the tympanic membrane. In J. Jerger (Ed.). *Modern developments in audiology.* New York, NY: Academic Press.

Margolis, R. H., & Goycoolea, H. G. (1993). Multifrequency tympanometry in normal adults. *Ear and Hearing, 14,* 408–413.

Margolis, R. H., & Hunter, L. L. (2002). Tympanometry—Basic principles and clinical application. In W. F. Rintlemann, & F. Musiek. (Eds.), *Contemporary perspectives on hearing assessment.* Boston, MA: Allyn & Bacon.

Margolis, R. H., Saly, G. L., & Keefe, D. H. (1999). Wideband reflectance tympanometry in normal adults. *Journal of the Acoustical Society of America, 106,* 265–280.

Margolis, R. H., & Smith, P. (1977). Tympanometric asymmetry. *Journal of Speech and Hearing Research, 20,* 437–446.

Margolis, R. H., Van Camp, K. J., Wilson, R. H., & Creten, W. L. (1985). Multifrequency tympanometry in normal ears. *Audiology, 24,* 44–53.

Maw, A. R., & Bawden, R. (1994). Tympanic membrane atrophy, scarring, atelectasis and attic retraction in persistent, untreated otitis media with effusion and following ventilation tube insertion. *International Journal of Pediatric Otorhinolaryngology, 30,* 189–204.

Merchant, G. R., Horton, N. J., & Voss, S. E. (2010). Normative reflectance and transmittance measurements on healthy newborn and 1-month-old infants. *Ear and Hearing, 31,* 746–754.

Miani, C., Bergamin, A. M., Barotti, A., & Isola, M. (2000). Multifrequency multicomponent tympanometry in normal and otosclerotic ears. *Scandinavian Audiology, 29,* 225–237.

Muchnik, C., Hildesheimer, M., Rubinstein, M., & Glettman, Y. (1989). Validity of tympanometry in cases of confirmed otosclerosis. *Journal of Laryngology and Otology, 103,* 36–38.

Newby, H. A., & Popelka, G. R. (1992). *Audiology* (6th ed.). Englewood Cliffs, NJ: Prentice-Hall.

Shahnaz, N., Bork, K., Polka, L., Longridge, N., Bell, D., & Westerberg, B. D. (2009). Energy reflectance and tympanometry in normal and otosclerotic ears. *Ear and Hearing, 30,* 219–233.

Shahnaz, N., & Davies, D. (2006). Standard and multifrequency tympanometric norms for Caucasian and Chinese young adults. *Ear and Hearing, 27,* 75–90.

Shahnaz, N., Miranda, T., & Polka, L. (2008). Multifrequency tympanometry in neonatal intensive care unit and well babies. *Journal of the American Academy of Audiology, 19,* 392–418.

Shahnaz, N., & Polka, L. (1997). Standard and multifrequency tympanometry in normal and otosclerotic ears. *Ear and Hearing, 18,* 326–341.

Shahnaz, N., & Polka, L. (2002). Distinguishing healthy from otosclerotic ears: Effect of probe-tone frequency on static immittance. *Journal of the American Academy of Audiology, 13,* 345–355.

Shanks, J. E. (1984). Tympanometry. *Ear and Hearing, 5,* 268–280.

Shanks, J. E., Wilson, R. H., & Cambron, N. K. (1993). Multiple frequency tympanometry: Effects of ear canal volume compensation on static acoustic admittance and estimates of middle ear resonance. *Journal of Speech and Hearing Research, 36,* 178–185.

Valvik, B. R., Johnsen, M., & Laukli, E. (1994). Multifrequency tympanometry. *Audiology, 33,* 245–253.

Van Camp, K. J., Margolis, R. H., Wilson, R. H., Creten, W. L., & Shanks, J. E. (1986). Principles of tympanometry. *ASHA Monographs, 24,* 1–88.

Van Camp, K. J., & Vogeleer, M. (1986). Normative multifrequency tympanometric data on otosclerosis. *Scandinavian Audiology, 15,* 187–190.

Vander Werff, K.R., Prieve, B.A., & Georgantas, L.M. (2007). Test-retest reliability of wideband reflectance measures in infants under screening and diagnostic test conditions. *Ear and Hearing, 28,* 669–681.

Vanhuyse, V. J., Creten, W. L., & Van Camp, K. J. (1975). On the W-notching of tympanograms. *Scandinavian Audiology, 4,* 45–50.

Wada, H., Kobayashi, T., Suetake, M., & Tachizaki, H. (1989). Dynamic behavior of the middle ear based on sweep frequency tympanometry. *Audiology, 28,* 127–134.

Wada, H., Koike, T., & Kobayashi, K. (1998). Clinical application of the sweep frequency measuring apparatus for diagnosis of middle ear diseases. *Ear and Hearing, 19,* 240–249.

Wiley, T. L., Cruickshanks, K. J., Nondahl, D. M., & Tweed, T. S. (1999). Aging and middle ear resonance. *Journal of the American Academy of Audiology, 10,* 173–179.

Yost, W. A. (2000). *Fundamentals of hearing.* San Diego, CA: Academic Press.

Zhao, F., Lowe, G., Meredith, R., & Rhodes, A. (2008). The characteristics of otoreflectance and its test-retest reliability. *Asia Pacific Journal of Speech, Language, and Hearing, 11,* 1–7.

Zhao, F., Meredith, R. N., Wotherspoon, N., & Rhodes, A. (2007, July). Towards an understanding of middle ear mechanism using otoreflectance: The characteristics of energy reflectance. *Proceedings of the 4th Symposium on Middle Ear Mechanics and Otology* (pp. 60–68). Zurich, Switzerland.

Zhao, F., Wada, H., Koike, T., Ohyama, K., Kawase, T., & Stephens, D. (2002). Middle ear dynamic characteristics in patients with otosclerosis. *Ear and Hearing, 23,* 150–158.

Zhao, F., Wada, H., Koike, T., Ohyama, K., Kawase, T., & Stephens, D. (2003). Transient evoked otoacoustic emissions in pa-tients with middle ear disorders. *International Journal of Audiology, 42,* 117–131.

Zwislocki, J. J. (1982). Normal function of the middle ear and its measurement. *Audiology, 21,* 4–14.

CHAPTER 6

Current Developments in the Clinical Application of the Sweep Frequency Impedance (SFI) in Assessing Middle Ear Dysfunction

MICHIO MURAKOSHI, FEI ZHAO, AND HIROSHI WADA

INTRODUCTION

The sweep frequency impedance (SFI) meter, developed in the 1990s, was designed to measure the middle ear dynamic characteristics of the middle ear in adults and children, (Wada & Kobayashi, 1990; Wada, Kobayashi, Suetake, & Tachizaki, 1989; Wada, Koike, & Kobayashi, 1998; Zhao, Wada, Koike, Ohyama, Kawase, & Stephens, 2002, 2003). The SFI utilizes a different approach from current multifrequency tympanometers in that it does not measure the admittance of the middle ear. Instead, it measures the sound pressure level in the ear canal when a stimulus with frequency varying from 0.1 to 2 kHz is delivered to the ear at various static applied air pressures. In this chapter, we start by providing background information on the engineering design and working principles of the SFI device. This is followed by presentation of normative data and discussion of current clinical applications using the SFI in adults, infants, and neonates.

ENGINEERING DESIGN AND MEASUREMENT PRINCIPLE OF THE SFI DEVICE

Functioning of the Apparatus

A block diagram of the SFI meter is shown in Figure 6–1. Measurement of the sound pressure level in the ear canal begins as the probe-tone frequency is swept from 0.1 kHz to 2.0 kHz in 4 s, whereas the external auditory meatus static pressure (P_s) is held constant. The measurements are performed with an initial applied pressure of 200 daPa down to −200 daPa at 50-daPa intervals. Measurements are also performed at the pressure point where the peak of the conventional tympanogram occurs. The sweeping probe tone is delivered to the external auditory meatus at a level below 80 dB SPL, which is below the stapedial reflex threshold. The sweeping tone is calibrated using a 2-cc coupler at a frequency of 1 kHz. The entire procedure for the automatic recording of results takes about 1 minute per ear.

The measured sound pressure is expressed by the differences in SPL (ΔSPL, in dB), and the phase (θ, in degrees) as shown by the following equations:

$$\Delta SPL = 20 \log \left| P/P_{REF} \right| \qquad \text{Eqn. (1)}$$

$$\theta = \tan^{-1}\left(\frac{-\text{Im}(P)}{\text{Re}(P)}\right) - \tan^{-1}\left(\frac{-\text{Im}(P_{REF})}{\text{Re}(P_{REF})}\right)$$

$$\text{Eqn. (2)}$$

where P is the sound pressure in the external ear canal, and Re(P) and Im(P) are the real and imaginary parts of P, respectively, and the subscript REF means the reference.

Frequency Characteristics of the Probe Tip

The frequency characteristics of the probe tip are measured in a calibration cavity, which is a plastic injector cylinder closed at one end. Measurement commences when the probe tip is inserted into the open end of the cylinder. The measurement results are depicted in Figure 6–2. The ΔSPL curves decrease

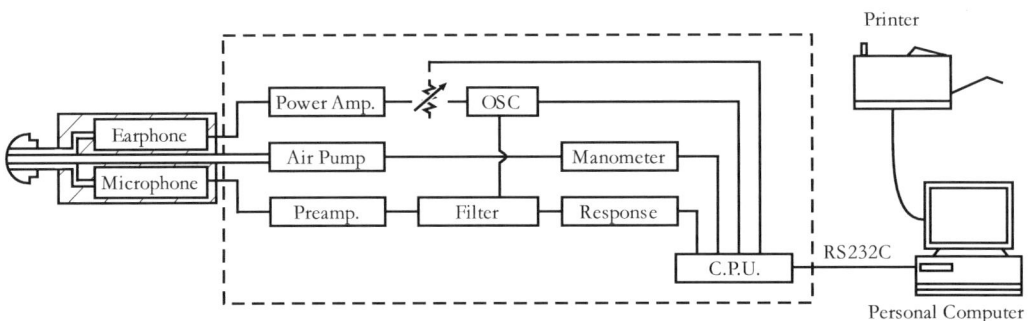

FIGURE 6–1. Block diagram of measurement apparatus. (From Wada et al. [1989]. *Ear and Hearing, 19,* 240–249. Copyright © 1998 by Williams & Wilkins. Reprinted by permission of Williams & Wilkins.)

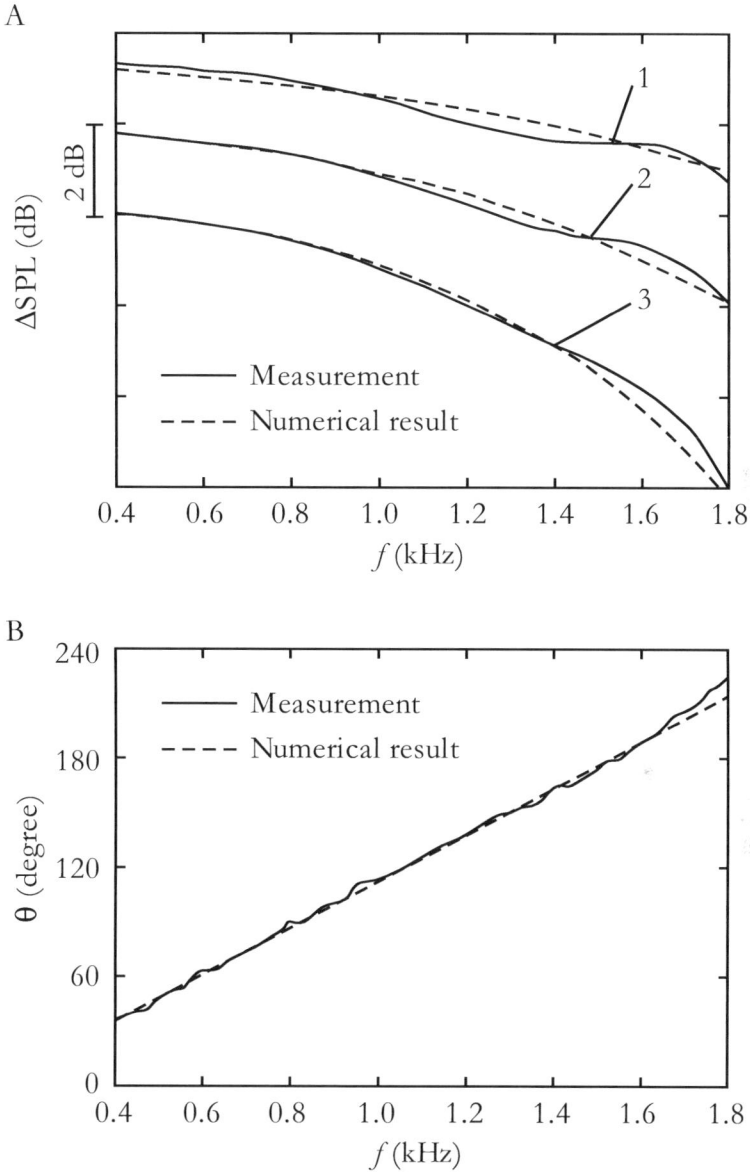

FIGURE 6–2. Measurement results of the calibration cavity. **A.** ΔSPL curves: 1, l_c = 3.0 cm; 2, l_c = 3.5 cm; 3, l_c = 4.0 cm. **B.** Phase $θ$ curves when P_s = 0 daPa and l_c = 3.5 cm. If the calibration cavity is a pure acoustic compliance, $θ$ = 0°. —, measurement; ----, numerical result. (From Wada and Kobayashi [1990]. *Journal of the Acoustical Society of America, 87*, 237–245. Copyright © 1990 by The Acoustical Society of America [ASA]. Reprinted by permission of American Institute of Physics [on behalf of ASA].)

gradually with an increase in the frequency, and the decrease ratio of ΔSPL is large when the length of the calibration cavity is large. The phase θ between the earphone and the microphone increases linearly with an increase in the frequency f, and the increase ratio of phase θ is independent of the length of the calibration cavity l_c between 3.0 and 4.0 cm. The effect of external auditory canal pressure P_s on the frequency characteristics of the probe tip is negligibly small (not shown here).

In Figures 6–2A and 6–2B, comparisons between measurement (experimental) results and theoretical values of ΔSPL and phase θ (taken from Wada & Kobayashi, 1988) are made. As shown, the numerical results are fairly coincident with the experimental ones. This means that the probe tip exhibits flat frequency characteristics. In Figure 6–2A, for the sake of clarity, the reference values at the frequency f = 0.4 kHz are altered appropriately.

SFI DATA FROM NORMAL ADULTS AND THEORETICAL CONSIDERATIONS

Measurement Data

Fifty normally hearing adults were examined using the SFI. Most of them were young university students. Figure 6–3 depicts typical measurement results of the dynamic characteristics of the middle ear of these subjects. The ΔSPL variation versus the frequency f as a parameter of the external auditory canal pressure P_s is shown in Figure 6–3A. When P_s = 0 daPa, the ΔSPL curve (Curve 1) shows a large variation in SPL between 0.8 and 1.0 kHz, which is considered to be the resonance frequency region of the middle ear (Wada & Kobayashi, 1990). The resonance frequency region increases and the variation ratio of ΔSPL decreases as the external auditory pressure P_s increases, and the ΔSPL curve decreases monotonously with an increase in the frequency when P_s = 100 daPa. This means that the eardrum vibration is almost completely suppressed by P_s when P_s > 100 daPa. As shown in Figure 6–3B, phase θ between the earphone and the microphone increases linearly with an increase in frequency f, except for the resonance frequency region. In Figure 6–3A, the reference values of ΔSPL at f = 0.4 kHz are altered appropriately for the sake of clarity. Although not all examples are shown here, our measurement reveals that the individual differences of the dynamic characteristics of the middle ear are large, even in normally hearing adults.

Theoretical Analysis

The model shown in Figure 6–4 is used to simulate the complicated configuration of the human middle ear (Donaldson & Miller, 1980). Its geometry and all of its parameters are the same as those reported by Wada and Kobayashi (1990). That is, a, l, S, and V mean the

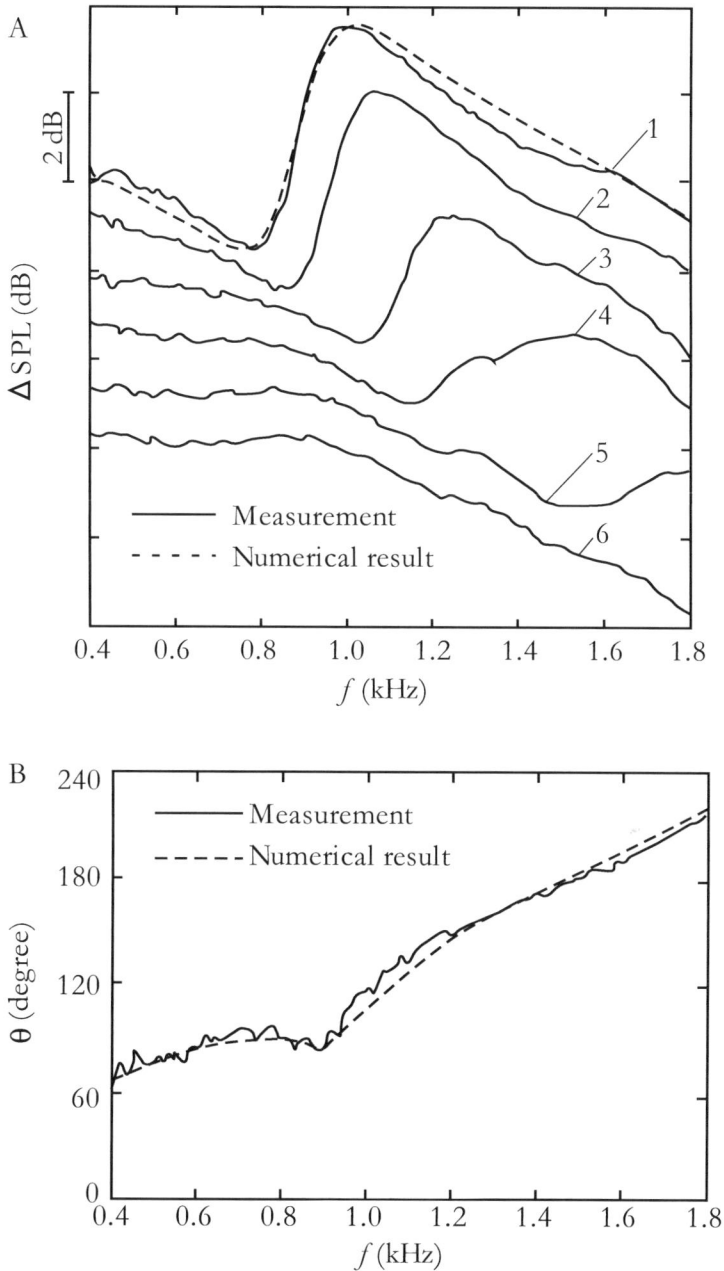

FIGURE 6–3. Typical measurement results in normal subjects. **A.** ΔSPL curves; 1, P_s = 0 daPa; 2, P_s = l0 daPa; 3, P_s = 20 daPa; 4, P_s = 30 daPa; 5, P_s = 50 daPa; 6, P_s = 100 daPa. **B.** Phase θ curves when P_s = 0 daPa. —, measurement; ----, numerical result. (From Wada and Kobayashi [1990]. *Journal of the Acoustical Society of America*, 87, 237–245. Copyright © 1990 by The Acoustical Society of America [ASA]. Reprinted by permission of American Institute of Physics [on behalf of ASA].)

Tympanic membrane Ossicular chain Tympanic cavity
(*TM*) (*O*) (*TC*)

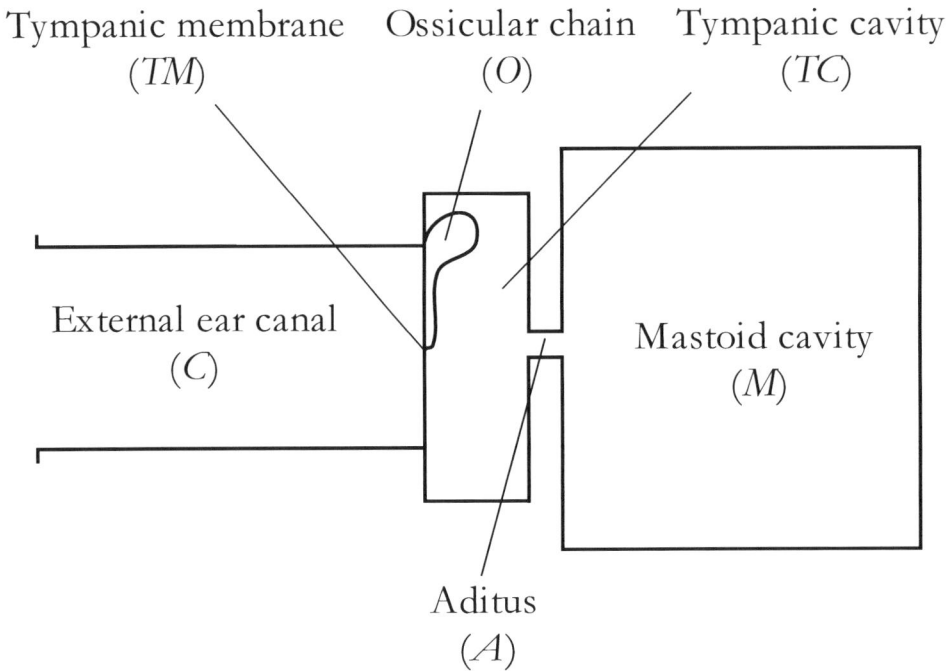

External ear canal
(*C*)

Mastoid cavity
(*M*)

Aditus
(*A*)

FIGURE 6–4. Analytical model of external and middle ears in humans. (From Wada and Kobayashi [1990]. *Journal of the Acoustical Society of America*, 87, 237–245. Copyright © 1990 by The Acoustical Society of America [ASA]. Reprinted by permission of American Institute of Physics [on behalf of ASA].)

radius, length, cross-sectional area, and volume, respectively. The subscripts *C, TM, O, TC, A,* and *M* stand for the external ear canal, tympanic membrane, ossicular chain, tympanic cavity, aditus, and mastoid cavity, respectively.

The relationship between the sound pressure *P* in the external ear canal and the constant volume displacement of a diaphragm of a speaker ΔV is given in the form:

$$\frac{P}{\Delta V} = j\omega \frac{Z_{ALL}\cos\gamma l_C + jS_C\rho_a u_a\sin\gamma l_C}{S_C^2[\cos\gamma l_C + jZ_{ALL}(1/S_C\rho_a u_a)\sin\gamma l_C]}$$

Eqn. (3)

where $u_a = (K_a^*/\rho_a)^{1/2}$ is the sound velocity,

$K_a^* = K_a(1 + j\eta\omega)$ and ρ_a are the complex bulk modulus and the density of the air, respectively. η is the air damping coefficient, $\omega = 2\pi f$ is the angular frequency, $\gamma = \omega/u_a$ is the wave number, $j = (-1)^{1/2}$, and Z_{ALL} is the mechanical impedance at the external ear canal side of the tympanic membrane.

If the volume displacement delivered from the earphone is constant over the frequency range 0.1 to 2.0 kHz, the measured sound pressure *P* at the microphone varies in conjunction with the variation of Z_{ALL}.

The mechanical impedance Z_{ALL} can be divided into three impedances in the form:

$$Z_{ALL} = Z_M + Z_{TM} + Z_O \qquad \text{Eqn. (4)}$$

where Z_M is the mechanical impedance of the middle-ear cavity (the tympanic cavity), aditus, and mastoid cavity, which is exerted on the tympanic membrane. Z_{TM} and Z_O are the mechanical impedances of the tympanic membrane itself and that of the ossicular chain, respectively, which are exerted on the tympanic membrane. Introducing the equivalent mass m, the spring constant k, and the damping constant c, the mechanical impedances Z_M, Z_{TM}, and Z_O can be expressed as:

$$Z_M = j\omega m_M + \frac{1}{j\omega} k_M + c_M,$$

$$Z_{TM} = j\omega m_{TM} + \frac{1}{j\omega} k_{TM} + c_{TM},$$

$$Z_O = j\omega m_O + \frac{1}{j\omega} k_O + c_O.$$

$$\text{Eqn. (5)}$$

As shown in Figure 6–4, when the cross-sections of the cavities change, the equivalent mass m_M, spring constant k_M, and damping constant c_M are derived from Hayasaka and Yoshikawa (1974) as:

$$m_M = \frac{S_{TM}^2}{S_{TC}} \frac{\rho_a\{(S_{TC}/S_A)l_A + (1+V_A/V_M)l_{TC}\}}{1 + V_A/V_M + V_{TC}/V_M},$$

$$k_M = \frac{S_{TM}^2}{S_{TC}} \frac{S_{TC}K_a/V_M}{1 + V_A/V_M + V_{TC}/V_M},$$

$$c_M = \frac{S_{TM}^2}{S_{TC}} \frac{\eta(S_{TC}K_a/V_M)}{1 + V_A/V_M + V_{TC}/V_M}.$$

$$\text{Eqn. (6)}$$

When the tympanic membrane vibrates under deflection due to the static pres-

sure applied to the external ear canal, the equivalent mass m_{TM}, spring constant k_{TM}, and damping constant c_{TM} of the tympanic membrane, and those of the ossicular chain, that is, m_{MO}, k_O, and c_O, can be obtained with the Lagrange equation as:

$$m_{TM} = \frac{9}{5} \rho_{TM} S_{TM} b_{TM},$$

$$m_O = \frac{9J}{a_{TM}^2},$$

$$k_{TM} = 18\alpha_{TM}\left(1 + \frac{6\beta_{TM}\Delta_S^2}{\alpha_{TM}}\right),$$

$$k_O = 18\alpha_O\left(1 + \frac{6\beta_O\Delta_S^2}{\alpha_O}\right),$$

$$c_{TM} = 2\xi_{TM}\sqrt{m_{TM}k_{TM}},$$

$$c_O = 2\xi_O\sqrt{m_O k_O},$$

$$\text{Eqn. (7)}$$

where

$$\alpha_{TM} = \frac{32}{3}\pi\frac{D_{TM}}{a_{TM}^2},$$

$$\alpha_O = \frac{M}{2a_{TM}^2},$$

$$\beta_{TM} = 2.59\pi\frac{D_{TM}}{(a_{TM}b_{TM})^2},$$

$$\beta_O = \frac{\kappa M}{2(a_{TM}b_{TM})^2}.$$

$$\text{Eqn. (8)}$$

In Equations (7) and (8), $D_{TM} = E_{TM}b_{TM}^3/12(1-v^2)$ is the flexural rigidity of the tympanic membrane; E_{TM}, b_{TM}, and v are Young's modulus, the thickness, and Poisson's ratio of the tympanic membrane, respectively; ρ_{TM} is the density of the tympanic membrane; J is the mass moment of inertia of the ossicular chain; Δ_S is the center deflection of the tympanic membrane due to the static pressure P_S; M and κ are the angular stiffness and the pressure-dependent coefficient of the ossicular chain, respectively; ξ_{TM} and ξ_O are the damping coefficient of the tympanic membrane and the ossicular chain, respectively.

The procedure for deriving the theoretical (numerical) values is as follows: First, the substitution of the values of the middle ear configuration, for example, the external auditory canal length l_c, into Equation (5), gives the value of Z_M; Second, substituting the value of the eardrum deflection due to the external auditory canal pressure P_s into Equations (7) and (8) provides the values of Z_E and Z_o; Third, substituting these determined values into Equation (4) gives the value of the mechanical mpedance Z_{ALL}; Finally, the differences in SPL, that is, ΔSPL, and the phase θ versus the frequency f and the external auditory canal pressure P_s can be determined by substituting the value of Z_{ALL} into Equations (1) to (3).

Comparison Between Measurement Data and Theoretical Data

For numerical calculations, the average values of the adult middle ear configuration are used, that is, external auditory canal radius $a_C = 0.45$ cm, eardrum radius $a_E = 0.45$ cm, eardrum thickness $b_E = 0.008$ cm (Uebo, Kodama, Oka, & Ishii, 1988), tympanic cavity volume V_τ = 0.5 cm³, aditus volume $V_A = 0.3 \times 10^{-2}$ cm³, and mastoid cavity volume $V_M = 2.0$ cm³. The external auditory canal length l_c is determined to be 3.5 cm from comparison between the measurement results of Figure 6–2 and that of Figure 6–3A when $P_s = 100$ daPa.

As the mechanical properties of the eardrum have not been well clarified (Funnell & Laszlo, 1982), these values were determined in our laboratory using the following procedure. First, the condition of only the eardrum attachment to the temporal bone of a fresh cadaver was made. Then, the ΔSPL curves of this specimen were measured using the SFI device. The measurement results were compared with the theoretically derived (numerical) values. The obtained values were as follows: eardrum density $\rho_E = 1.2$ g/cm³, eardrum Young's modulus $E_E = 3.3 \times 10^8$ dyn/cm², eardrum Poisson's ratio $v = 0.3$, and eardrum damping parameter $\xi_E = 0.16$. As the assumption of a flat circular eardrum was applied in the theoretical analysis, the actual value of the eardrum Young's modulus might have been smaller than the one obtained. The value of the mass moment of inertia of the ossicular chain J was determined to be $J = 0.7 \times 10^{-3}$ g·cm² from the weight and configuration of actual ossicular chain extracted from fresh cadavers. When determining the value of J, it was assumed that the two concentrated masses of the malleus head and the rest of the malleus rotate around its center of gravity (Kirikae, 1960). The mechanical properties of the ossicular chain are also very poorly understood (Funnell & Laszlo,

1982). Therefore, these values were determined from comparison between the numerical and measurement results to be the ossicular chain angular stiffness $M = 2.3 \times 10^4$ dyn·cm, the pressure-dependent coefficient $\kappa = 2.0$, and the ossicular chain-damping parameter $\xi_0 = 0.21$. The numerical results are shown in Figure 6–3 with broken line curves and Figure 6–5 with solid curves, which are fairly coincident with the measurement results shown in Figure 6–3.

CLINICAL APPLICATIONS OF THE SFI DEVICE IN ADULTS

Features of the SFI Data

The unique features of the SFI test are that more details of middle ear dynamic characteristics can be provided in two- and three-dimensional graphs (Figures 6–6 and 6–7), and, consequently, the resonance frequency and middle ear mobility

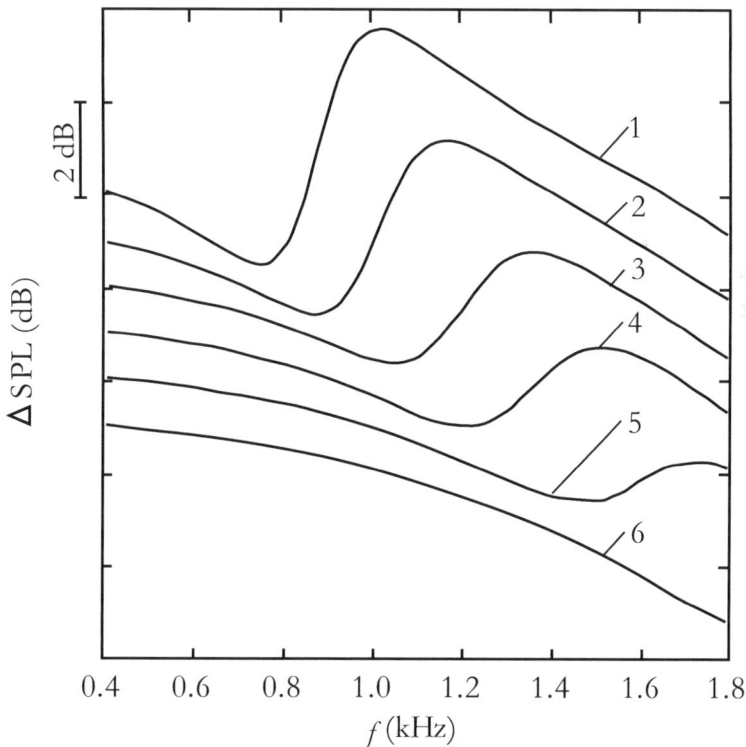

FIGURE 6–5. Numerical results. ΔSPL curves: 1, $P_s = 0$ daPa; 2, $P_s = 10$ daPa; 3, $P_s = 20$ daPa; 4, $P_s = 30$ daPa; 5, $P_s = 50$ daPa; 6, $P_s = 100$ daPa. (From Wada and Kobayashi [1990]. *Journal of the Acoustical Society of America, 87,* 237–245. Copyright © 1990 by The Acoustical Society of America [ASA]. Reprinted by permission of American Institute of Physics [on behalf of ASA].)

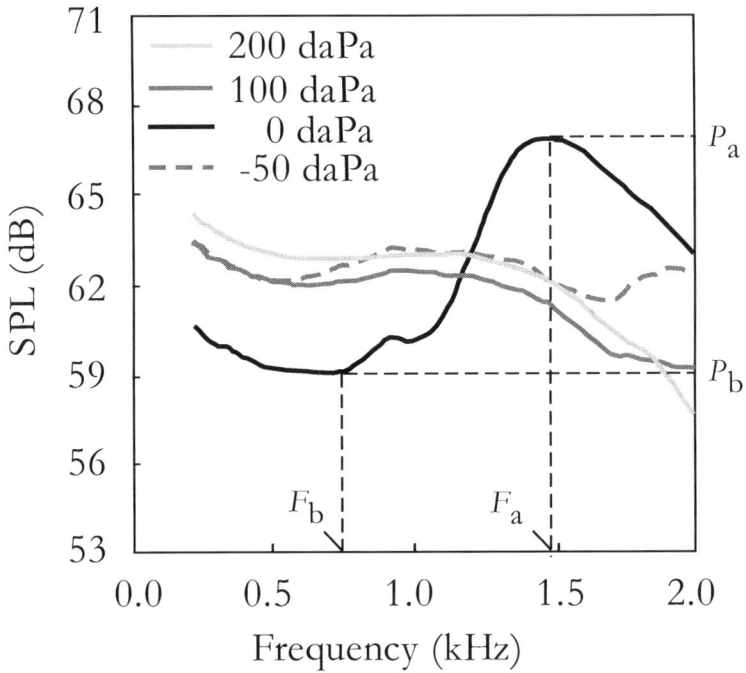

FIGURE 6–6. An example of the SFI results represented by a two-dimensional graph.

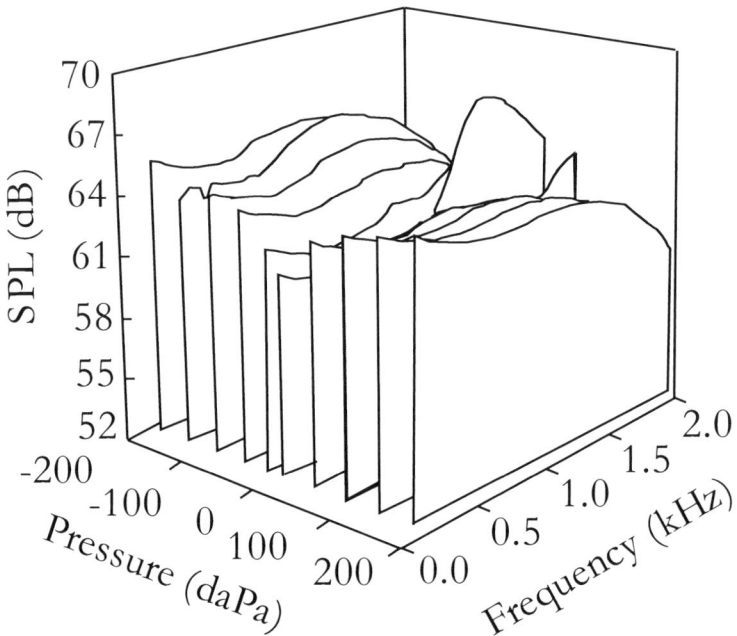

FIGURE 6–7. An example of the SFI results shown by a three-dimensional graph.

in terms of sound pressure change (ΔSPL) can be measured directly.

As shown in Figure 6–6, the maximum and minimum sound pressures (i.e., P_a and P_b) as well as the frequencies corresponding to these sound pressures (i.e., F_a and F_b) are chosen from visual inspection by testers (they could also be calculated using an automated mathematical procedure after converting all data to a digital format). Once these points are monitored using cursors, both resonance frequency and ΔSPL are automatically calculated using the following equations:

$$\text{Resonance frequency} = (F_a + F_b)/2$$
Eqn. (9)

$$\Delta SPL = P_a - P_b \qquad \text{Eqn. (10)}$$

Although the ΔSPL is considered to be an index of middle ear mobility, it varies as the resonance frequency shifts from low toward high frequency (see Figure 6–5). When the resonance frequency is toward the higher frequency region (e.g., close to 2.0 kHz), the ΔSPL tends to decrease. In contrast, when the resonance frequency is toward the lower frequency region, the ΔSPL value increases. At extreme pressures (i.e., P_s = ±200 daPa), the sound-pressure curves uniformly decrease with an increase in the frequency f with no peak identified, indicating that the resonance frequency may be greater than 2 kHz.

From a three-dimensional perspective, the resonance frequency increases and the value of the ΔSPL decreases as the static pressure of the external auditory meatus is increased from −200 to 200 daPa. This relationship among sound pressure changes, probe frequency f and the external auditory meatus static pressure P_s, is clearly shown in Figure 6–7. It provides information on the middle ear dynamic characteristics, including the resonance frequency and the sound pressure change (ΔSPL), which reflects the magnitude of the tympanic membrane volume displacement at the resonance frequency and the mobility of the middle ear.

SFI Data for Normal-Hearing Subjects

The normative data for adults have been published in studies by Wada et al. (1998) and Zhao et al. (2003). In the study by Wada et al. (1998), the authors measured 275 ears with intact tympanic membrane and normal hearing using the SFI device. Figure 6–8A depicts typical measurement results of a normal-hearing subject. As described previously, when the static pressure is not applied to the external auditory meatus (P_s = 0 daPa), the sound pressure curve varies considerably in the frequency region around 1.2 kHz. This frequency region is considered to be the resonance frequency region of the middle ear, and the pressure difference between the bottom of the curve and its peak reflects the magnitude of the tympanic membrane volume displacement at the resonance frequency (Wada, Ohyama, Kobayashi, Sunaga, & Koike, 1993). When the value of the ΔSPL is large, the tympanic membrane volume displacement is large and vice versa.

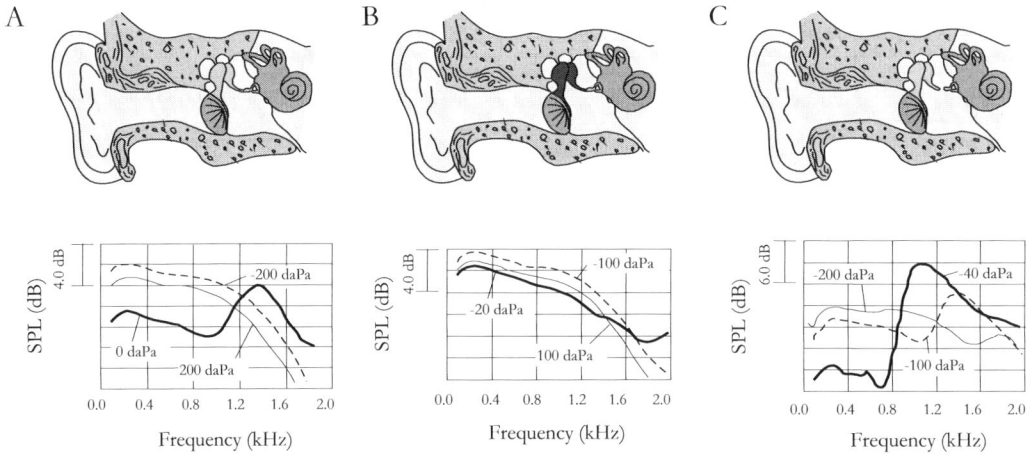

FIGURE 6–8. Typical results of SFI measurement. **A.** Normal-hearing subject. **B.** Patient with ossicular chain fixation. **C.** Patient with ossicular chain separation. Based on the results of (A), the middle ear resonance frequency is 1.2 kHz when the external auditory meatus static pressure P_s is 0 daPa.

Ossicular Chain Fixation

Figure 6–8B shows representative measurement results of a patient with ossicular chain fixation. The static compliance, as measured using conventional tympanometry, was 0.28 mL. Surgery revealed that the tympanic membrane and ossicles of this patient were normal but that the stapedius muscle was ossified. When P_s is −20 daPa, a small ΔSPL is observed at 1.8 kHz. This frequency is higher than that of a normal-hearing subject. The resonance frequency region disappears when a slight static pressure is applied to the external auditory meatus. These results are similar to those obtained from patients with malleus and/or incus fixation. In general, the following characteristics are observed in patients with typical ossicular chain fixation: (1) The resonance frequency is higher than that of a normal-hearing subject; (2) The value of the ΔSPL is smaller than that of a normal-hearing subject; and (3) The effects of the external auditory meatus pressure on the middle ear dynamic characteristics are larger than those of a normal-hearing subject.

Zhao et al. (2002) conducted a study on patients with otosclerosis using the SFI device. Various middle ear dynamic characteristics were observed depending on the different pathologic stages involving the stapes footplate. High resonance frequency and low ΔSPL were found in 44.4% (16/36) of the otosclerotic ears. The SFI findings are consistent with abnormally high stiffness of the middle ear system. When the outcomes of the SFI and conventional tympanometry were compared, a significantly higher percentage of abnormal stiffness was found when using the SFI test than when using conventional tympanometry. This confirms the advantage of the SFI test over conventional tympanometry in identifying patients with otosclerosis. Moreover, different middle ear dynamic characteristics in patients with otosclerosis are most likely to be related to the different stages of the pathological changes.

Ossicular Chain Separation

When compared with results obtained from normal ears, the SFI findings for ears with ossicular chain separation showed a lower resonance frequency and increased ΔSPL. These characteristic results indicate a low-stiffness middle ear system (Wada et al., 1998; Zhao et al., 2003). Figure 6–8C shows representative measurement results of a patient with incudostapedial joint separation. The static compliance is 1.50 mL, which is within the 90% range for normal adults (Roup, Wiley, Safady, & Stoppenbach, 1998). The results of this patient are clearly different from those of normal-hearing subjects. The resonance frequency is 0.66 kHz when P_s is 0 daPa, which is lower than the typical measurement result of normal-hearing subjects shown in Figure 6–8A. The value of the ΔSPL is 18.8 dB, which is three times larger than the normal value. As the static pressure decreases to −40 daPa, the resonance frequency increases and ΔSPL decreases. However, the rate of these changes is smaller than that of normal-hearing subjects. At P_s = −200 daPa, the sound-pressure variation due to resonance can still be observed, although this variation is not observed in normal-hearing subjects.

In summary, the qualitative characteristics of SFI results obtained from patients with typical ossicular chain separation are: (1) The resonance frequency is lower than that of a normal-hearing subject; (2) The value of the ΔSPL is larger than that of a normal-hearing subject; and (3) The effects of the external auditory meatus static pressure on the middle ear dynamic characteristics are smaller than those of a normal-hearing subject.

Otitis Media with Effusion

For patients with mild otitis media with effusion (OME), the SFI results show relatively normal middle ear dynamic characteristics in spite of a slightly negative pressure (−100 daPa tympanic peak pressure). The resonance frequency shifts slightly to high frequencies, together with a slightly reduced ΔSPL value at static pressure. However, in patients with severe secretory otitis media (SOM), the SFI findings indicate a high-stiffness middle ear with the resonance frequency being higher and ΔSPL reduced when compared to those of normally hearing adults (Wada et al., 1998; Zhao et al., 2003).

Tympanic Membrane Aberrations and Perforation

Wada et al. (1998) and Zhao et al. (2003) investigated the middle ear dynamic characteristics in patients with middle ear disorders using the SFI. Their results indicated that in patients with minor

TM scarring, the resonance frequency shifted slightly to high frequencies, together with a reduced ΔSPL value at the static pressure. These results indicate normal or close to normal middle ear dynamic characteristics. However, the SFI results in patients with retracted TM and tympanosclerosis indicated high resonance frequency with significantly reduced ΔSPL, consistent with a high-stiffness middle ear system. In patients with TM perforation, the sound-pressure variation is larger than that of a normal-hearing subject. In addition, a frequency notch was found in the area below 1.0 kHz.

GROUP SFI FINDINGS

The measurement results mentioned above show that the resonance frequency and value of the ΔSPL in patients differ from those of normal-hearing subjects. Table 6–1 summarizes the mean values and standard deviations of the resonance frequency, and the value of ΔSPL obtained from normal-hearing subjects (normal group), patients with ossicular chain separation (separation group) and patients with ossicular chain fixation (fixation group). The ossicular condition of the patients was confirmed by surgery. These mean values and standard deviations were calculated on the assumption that the resonance frequency and the logarithmic value of the ΔSPL have normal distributions. There were significant differences in the mean values of the resonance frequency and ΔSPL between the separation group and the fixation group ($p < 0.005$). The separation group had a low resonance frequency and large ΔSPL in comparison with the normal group. However, the differences between the normal group and the fixation group were small.

Figure 6–9A shows the distribution of the resonance frequency against ΔSPL for all three groups. Figure 6–9B shows a clear distribution map using spline curves to enclose the regions bound by the confidence intervals at

TABLE 6–1. Number of Subjects and Mean Values of Resonance Frequency and ΔSPL

		Normal	Separation	Fixation
	Subjects	153 (275 ears)	24 (26 ears)	12 (12 ears)
Resonance frequency (kHz)	Mean ± SD	1.17 ± 0.27	0.83 ± 0.25	1.40 ± 0.33
ΔSPL (dB)	Mean ± SD	2.18 ± 3.84	10.69 ± 4.51	1.37 ± 2.86

SD = standard deviation; *$p < 0.01$; **$p < 0.005$.

the 0.95 level for both the resonance frequency and ΔSPL. Although the three regions overlap each other, the region of the separation group differs from that of the fixation group.

Table 6–2 summarizes test results on 51 ears with ossicular chain patholo-gies. All pathologies were verified by surgery. The distribution of the types of the conventional 220 Hz tympanograms obtained from these ears is also shown in Table 6–2. The criterion for discrimi-nating Type A_D and A_s from Type A was based on a study by Ichimura, Kodera,

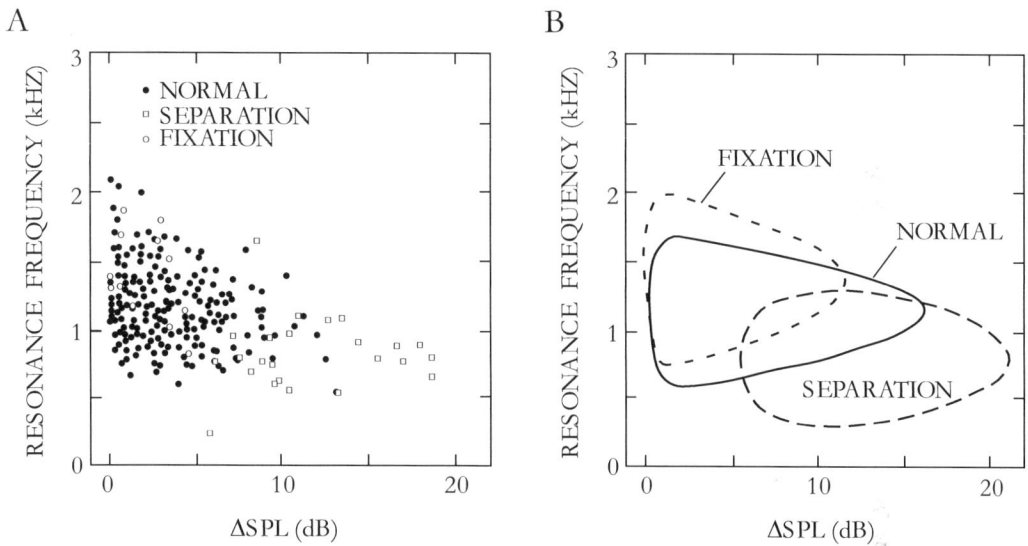

FIGURE 6–9. Distribution of measurement data of normal-hearing subjects and of patients. **A**. Measurement data are plotted on the resonance frequency-ΔSPL plane. **B**. Distribution map of middle ear dynamic characteristics. The confidence intervals at the 0.95 level for the resonance frequency and the value of ΔSPL are enclosed by spline curves. (From Wada et al. [1989]. *Ear and Hearing, 19*, 240–249. Copyright © 1998 by Williams & Wilkins. Reprinted by permission of Williams & Wilkins.)

TABLE 6–2. Diagnostic Results in Ears with Ossicular Chain Pathologies and Distribution of the Types of 220-Hz Tympanograms

Pathology	Diagnosis			Distribution				
	Ears	Correct	False	Ears	A_D	A	A_S	B
Separation	32	27 (84%)	5	29	15	13	1	0
Fixation	19	14 (74%)	5	19	0	9	4	6
Total	51	41 (80%)	10	48				

Type A_D = SC ≥ 1.22 mL; Type A = 0.23 mL < SC < 1.22 mL; Type A_S = SC ≤ 0.23 mL.

and Funasaka (1976). Out of the 32 ears with ossicular chain separation, 27 ears were correctly diagnosed based on the SFI diagnostic procedure, indicating a sensitivity of 84%. Fourteen out of the 19 ears were diagnosed correctly with ossicular chain fixation with a sensitivity of 74%. In contrast, the corresponding conventional 220-Hz tympanometric results showed Type A_D tympanograms in 15 out of the 29 ears with ossicular chain separation with a sensitivity of 52%. One ear with ossicular chain separation resulted in Type A_s instead of Type A_D. Tympanometry could not be performed on three ears because of a pressure leak. Out of the 19 ears with ossicular chain fixation, 9 ears (47%) showed Type A, 4 ears (21%) showed Type A_s and 6 ears (32%) showed Type B tympanograms.

Aging Effect on the Middle Ear Mobility

Two hundred and sixty-four ears of 160 normally hearing subjects ranging in age from 5 to 79 years were examined. The subjects were divided into eight groups by age. The relationship between ΔSPL (an indicator of middle ear mobility) and age is shown in Figure 6–10. In Figure 6–10A, all the measurement results are plotted with filled circles and open circles representing the data from males and females, respectively. In Figure 6–10B, the mean ΔSPL values of ± one standard deviation for males and females are plotted with solid and broken lines, respectively,

against age. Figure 6–10A shows that the ΔSPL values of the subjects were variable irrespective of age. As shown in Figure 6–10B, the mean ΔSPL values for males reached a maximum value of 3.1 dB between 10 and 20 years of age, then decreased slightly, reaching a plateau beyond 40 and 50 years of age. On the contrary, the mean value for females tended to increase with increasing age. Despite the variations in mean ΔSPL across gender and age, the differences were not statistically significant between 5-year-old children and adults due to large standard deviation values for these groups.

DEVELOPMENT OF THE SFI DEVICE FOR USE WITH INFANTS AND NEONATES

Although the SFI device has been used successfully to detect middle ear problems in adults, its application to infants (within a few years of age) and neonates (within 5 days of age) has never been explored until recently. The SFI device has recently been modified to enable it to be used with infants and neonates. A schematic diagram of the device is shown in Figure 6–11. The SFI device consists of a probe system, a syringe pump, a stepping motor, a pressure sensor, an AD/DA converter, and a personal computer. A schema and a photograph of this improved SFI meter are shown in Figures 6–11A and 6–11B, respectively.

To measure the dynamic characteristics of the middle ear in infants and

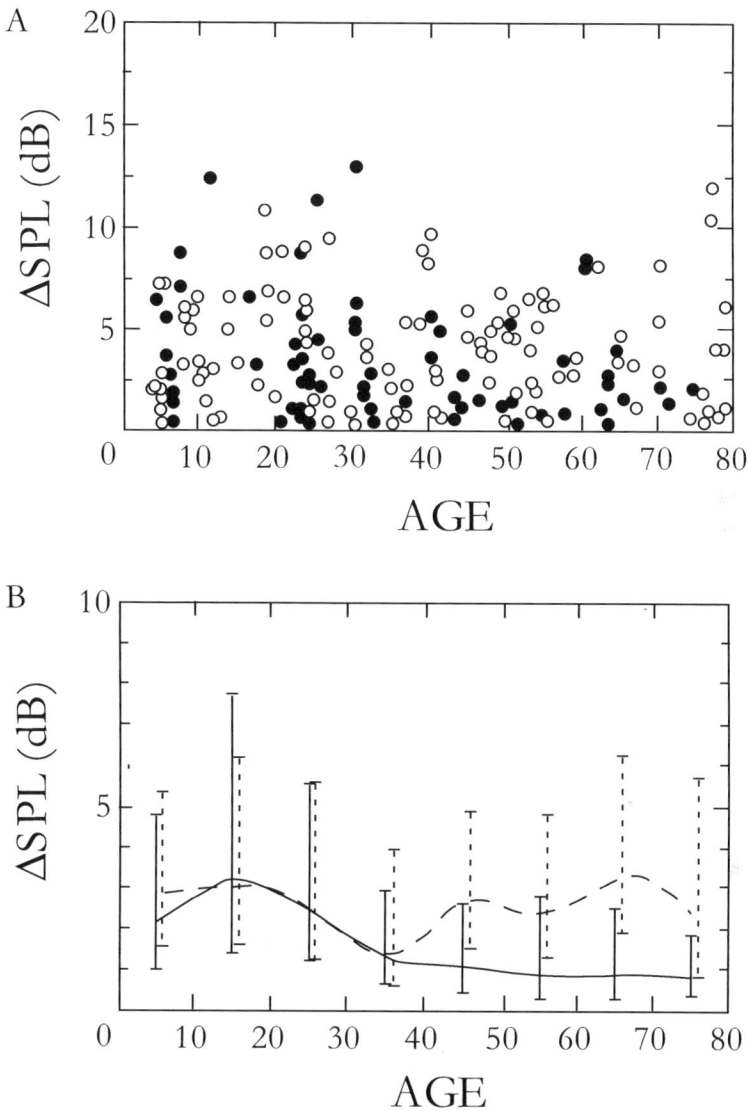

FIGURE 6–10. Relationship between the value of ΔSPL and age.
A. Filled circles and open circles represent the data on males and
females, respectively. **B**. Mean male and female ΔSPL values of
each group are plotted with solid and broken lines, respectively.
The vertical bars indicate one standard deviation from the mean.

neonates, the SFI probe was re-designed. Figure 6–12 shows a photograph of a new probe for infants and neonates, and the conventional probe for adults. As shown in Figure 6–12, the shape of the new probe is smaller than that of the conventional one. The diameter of the new probe is approximately 3 mm,

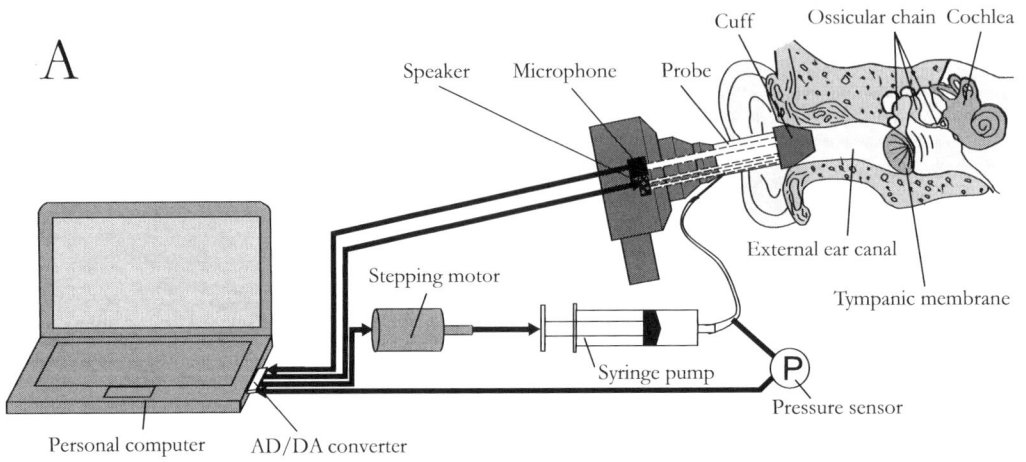

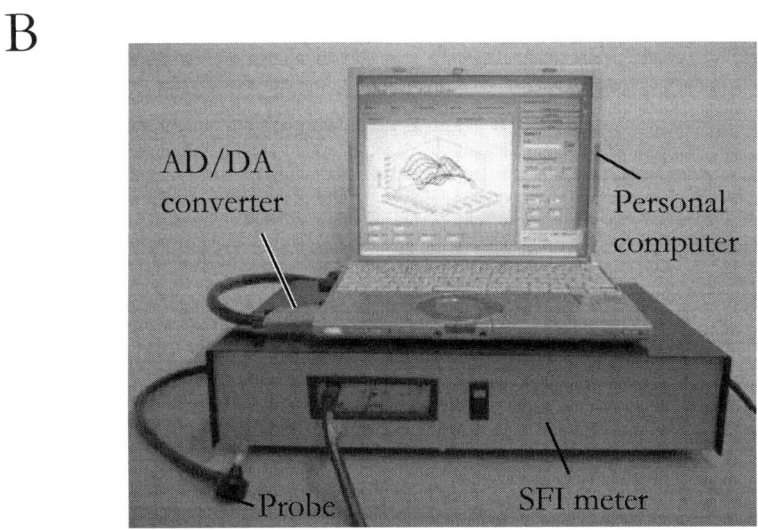

FIGURE 6–11. New SFI meter for testing infants and neonates. **A.** A schema of the SFI meter which consists of a probe system, a syringe pump, a stepping motor, a pressure sensor, an AD/DA converter, and a personal computer. This new SFI meter is controlled using LabView under WINDOWS. **B.** A photo of the new SFI meter setup.

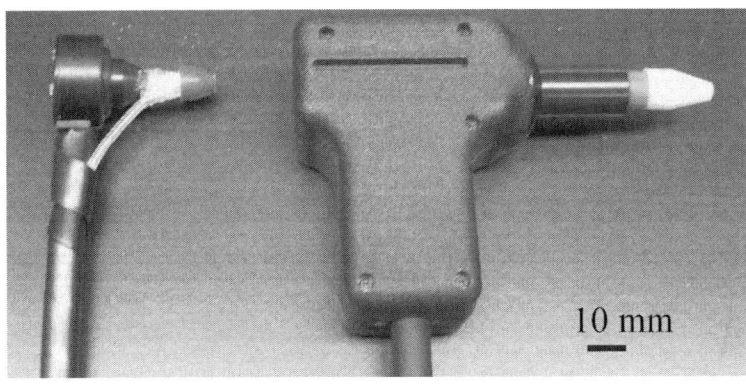

FIGURE 6–12. The SFI probes. Left—new probe for testing infants and neonates; Right—conventional probe for testing children and adults.

whereas that of the conventional probe is approximately 5 mm. There are three holes in this 3-mm probe: one for applying static pressure; one for delivering sound to the external ear canal; and the remaining one for measuring sound pressure using a microphone. A specially designed cuff suitable for testing infants and neonates is attached to the tip of the probe to seal off the ear canal during testing.

Preliminary SFI Findings in Neonates

Figure 6–13 shows a comparison of SFI results obtained from a normally hearing adult and a healthy neonate. As shown in Figure 6–13A, the sound pressure for the adult varies greatly at the frequency between 1.2 and 1.6 kHz, being the resonance frequency of the middle ear, at $P_s = -2$ daPa. The resonance frequency increases and the variation ratio of ΔSPL decreases as P_s increases. When P_s is larger than about ±100 daPa, the ΔSPL curve decreases monotonically with increasing frequency f.

Interestingly, the SFI results for the healthy neonate (as shown in Figure 6–13B) do not resemble the results for the normally hearing adult. When the static pressure in the external ear canal P_s was −1 daPa, the sound pressure varied greatly at around 0.3 kHz and 1.2 kHz. Such variations were still observed when P_s was 99 daPa. On the other hand, when a negative static pressure was applied to the external ear canal (e.g., $P_s = -102$ daPa), the ΔSPL curve did not show such variations.

Given the differences in SFI results between an adult and a neonate, the interpretation of the SFI results obtained from a neonate require special consideration. First, the number of the variations in the ΔSPL curve was different. In the measurement results for the neonate, two variations in the sound pressure were observed around 0.3 and 1.2 kHz. This result suggests that there are two vibrating elements in the neonatal external and middle ear. One of the vibrating elements which occurs around $f = 1.2$ kHz may be related to the resonance of the middle ear (Wada & Kobayashi, 1990). The other vibrating element which occurs around 0.3 kHz may be associated with the neonatal external ear canal, being more elastic than that of the adult (Qui, Liu, Lutfy, Funnell, & Daniel, 2006). This finding appears to be in line with the results obtained by Holte, Margolis, and Cavanaugh (1991) who found a resonance of around 0.45 kHz in a healthy neonate. This resonance must not be confused with the fundamental resonance frequency of the ear canal which varies from 5.3 to 7.2 kHz in children from birth to 3 years of age (Kruger, 1987).

EARLY CLINICAL TRIALS USING THE SFI DEVICE WITH NEONATES

Figure 6–14 shows the SFI results obtained from a normal-hearing neonate. The data shows two variations of the sound pressure at around 0.3 kHz and 1.2 kHz. Regarding the first variation,

A

B

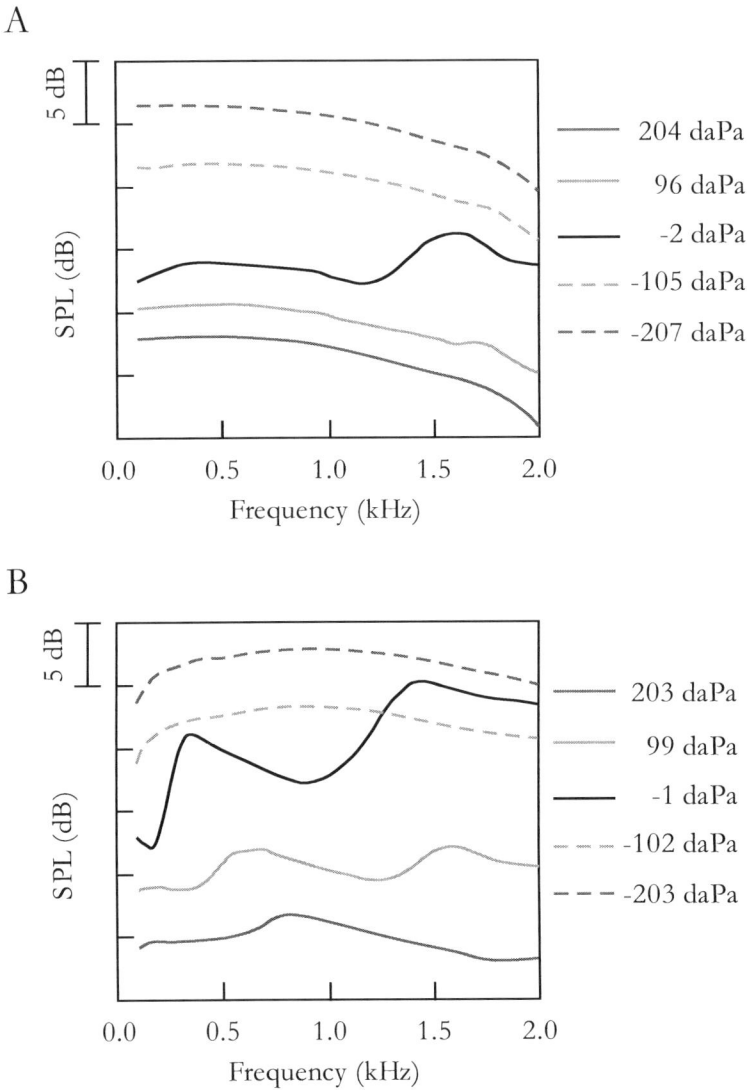

FIGURE 6–13. Representative SFI results for (**A**) a normally hearing adult; (**B**) a healthy neonate. When the static pressure applied to the external ear canal was near ambient pressure (about 0 daPa), two variations in the sound pressure were observed at around 0.3 kHz and 1.2 kHz for the neonate, whereas one variation was observed at 1.2 kHz for the adult. For clarity, the SPL curves were positioned in parallel to distinguish SPL curves.

the frequency at which this occurred was shifted toward a higher frequency when both positive and negative pressures were applied to the external audi-tory meatus. In addition, ΔSPL decreased with an increase in the absolute value of the static pressure applied to the external ear canal P_s.

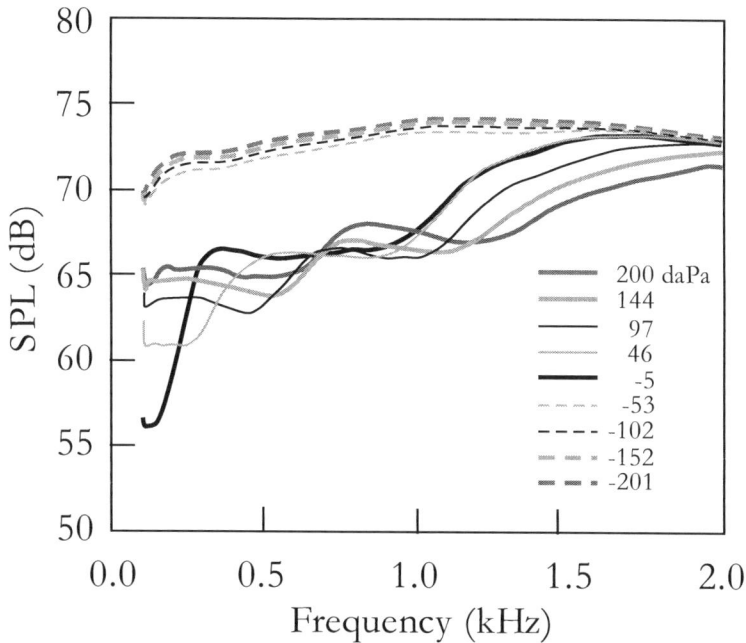

FIGURE 6–14. SFI results obtained from a normal-hearing neonate. The SPL curve at –5 daPa shows two variations in sound pressure, one at around 0.3 kHz and the other at 1.2 kHz.

Regarding the second variation which appeared at about 1.2 kHz when P_s = –5 daPa, it was in agreement with that reported in adults (Wada & Kobayashi, 1990), although the value of the ΔSPL was relatively larger (~10 dB) than that of normal-hearing adults (2.18 $\pm$ 3.84 dB; Wada et al., 1998). When a positive pressure was applied, the resonance shifted toward a higher frequency. The effects of the external auditory meatus static pressure on the variations in the sound pressure were smaller than those in normal-hearing adults; that is, the variations were still observed when the higher pressures of 200 daPa were applied. When the negative pressure became –53 daPa, ΔSPLs suddenly disappeared and showed flat responses with an increase in frequency. These results were consistent with the response observed using a calibration cavity, suggesting that the external ear canal might have collapsed under the negative pressure.

Figure 6–15 shows the SFI results obtained from a neonate with low middle-ear mobility, having failed the TEOAE, 1-kHz tympanometry, and acoustic stapedial reflex tests. The first variation in the sound pressure was observed at around 0.3 kHz; however, the second variation disappeared, suggesting middle ear dysfunction. Taken together, these findings suggest that the first and second variations possibly may be related to the resonance of the external and middle ears, respectively.

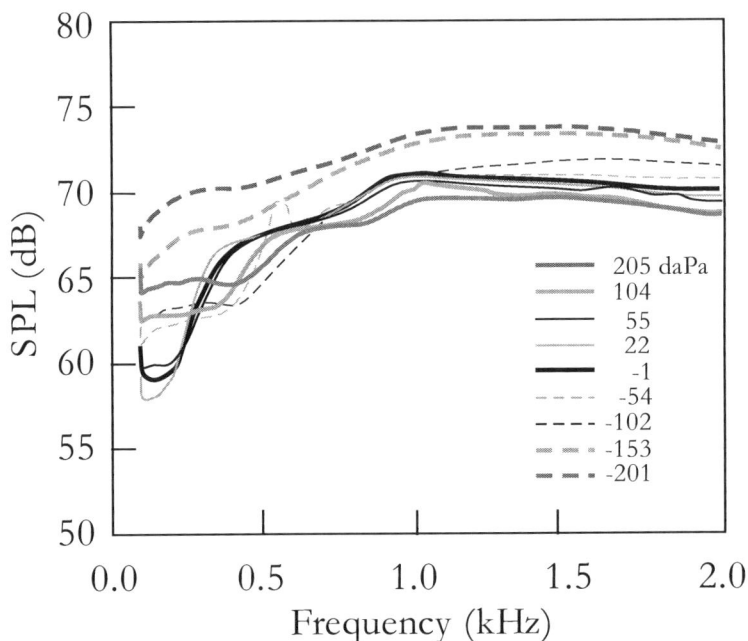

FIGURE 6–15. SFI result obtained from a neonate who failed the TEOAE, 1-kHz tympanometry, and acoustic stapedial reflex tests.

As this study was the first attempt to apply SFI measurement in neonates, further data and analysis will be required to clarify the detailed relationships between SFI results and the external and middle ear conditions.

REFERENCES

Donaldson, J. A., & Miller, J. M. (1980). *Anatomy of the Ear in Otolaryngology* (pp. 26–42). Philadelphia, PA: Saunders.

Funnell, W. R., & Laszlo, C. A. (1982). A critical review of experimental observations on ear-drum structure and function. *ORL: Journal for Oto-Rhino-Laryngology and Its Related Specialties*, *44*, 181–205.

Hayasaka, T., & Yoshikawa, S. (1974). *Acoustic vibration* [in Japanese]. Tokyo, Japan: Maruzen.

Holte, L., Margolis., R. H., & Cavanaugh, R. M. (1991). Developmental change in multifrequency tympanograms. *Audiology*, *30*, 1–24.

Ichimura, K., Kodera, K., & Funasaka, S. (1976). Impedance audiometry—its clinical application and diagnostic standard. *Journal of Otolaryngology*, *79*, 555–567 (in Japanese).

Kirikae, I. (1960). *The structural and function of the middle ear*. Tokyo, Japan: Tokyo University Press.

Kruger, B. (1987). An update on the external ear resonance in infants and young children. *Ear and Hearing*, *8*(6), 333–336.

Qui, L., Liu, H., Lutfy, J., Funnell, W. R., & Daniel, S. J. (2006). A nonlinear finite-element model of the newborn ear canal. *Journal of the Acoustical Society of America*, *120*, 3789–3798.

Roup, C. M., Wiley, T. L., Safady, S. H., & Stoppenbach, D. T. (1998). Tympanometry screening norms for adults. *American Journal of Audiology, 7,* 55–60.

Uebo, K., Kodama, A., Oka, Y., & Ishii, T. (1988). Thickness of normal human tympanic membrane [in Japanese]. *Ear Research Japan, 19,* 70–73.

Wada, H., & Kobayashi, T. (1988). Analysis of dynamical characteristics of middle ear: Theoretical study of three-dimensional tympanometry [in Japanese]. *Transactions of the Japan Society of Mechanical Engineers, 54,* 1671–1677.

Wada, H., & Kobayashi, T. (1990). Dynamical behavior of middle ear: Theoretical study corresponding to measurement results obtained by a newly developed measuring apparatus. *Journal of the Acoustical Society of America, 87,* 237–245.

Wada, H., Kobayashi, T., Suetake, M., & Tachizaki, H. (1989). Dynamic behavior of middle ear based on sweep frequency tympanometry. *Audiology, 28,* 127–134.

Wada, H., Koike, T., & Kobayashi, T. (1998). Clinical applicability of the sweep frequency measuring apparatus for diagnosis of middle ear diseases. *Ear and Hearing, 19,* 240–249.

Wada, H., Ohyama, K., Kobayashi, T., Sunaga, N., & Koike, T. (1993). Relationship between evoked otoacoustic emissions and middle ear dynamic characteristics. *Audiology, 32,* 282–292.

Zhao, F., Wada, H., Koike, T., Ohyama, K., Kawase, T., & Stephens, D. (2002). Middle ear dynamic characteristics in patients with otosclerosis. *Ear and Hearing, 23,* 150–158.

Zhao, F., Wada, H., Koike, T., Ohyama, K., Kawase, T., & Stephens, D. (2003). Transient evoked otoacoustic emissions in patients with middle ear disorders. *International Journal of Audiology, 42,* 117–131.

CHAPTER 7

Application of Wideband Acoustic Transfer Functions to the Assessment of the Infant Ear

M. PATRICK FEENEY AND CHRIS A. SANFORD

INTRODUCTION

This chapter introduces the concept of wideband acoustic transfer functions (ATFs) for the measurement of middle ear function. This approach to middle ear measurement, which has been developed over the last 2 to 3 decades, is beginning to prove remarkably useful for measurements in infant ears. In part, wideband ATFs are attractive because they extend the frequency region over which we can measure middle ear function to include the bandwidth of speech. The extended bandwidth is also proving useful in separating infant ears with middle ear disorders from those with normal middle ear function. Moreover, the application of power-based measures, which address the efficiency of the middle ear at acoustic power transfer, provide additional information to supplement and perhaps surpass the traditional immittance measures of admittance and impedance.

The chapter begins with a brief overview of the principles of wideband ATF measurement, followed by data on adults with normal middle ear function and adults with middle ear disorders, as well as acoustic stapedial reflex measurement. The second half of the chapter examines the application of wideband ATFs to the evaluation of the infant middle ear.

PRINCIPLES OF WIDEBAND ATFS FOR THE ANALYSIS OF MIDDLE EAR FUNCTION

The introduction of the term "immittance" for measures of middle ear function allowed the grouping of acoustic impedance and acoustic admittance measures into one category (ANSI 1987). Although acoustic impedance measurements have not found favor for commercial immittance systems, admittance tympanometry, and acoustic stapedial reflex measures using a 0.226-kHz probe tone have been used successfully in adults to evaluate middle ear function. However, these techniques have not been successfully used to evaluate middle ear function in infants less than 6 months of age (see Chapter 2 for a review). Keefe and Feeney (2009) suggested an expansion of the definition of immittance to consider the family of acoustic transfer functions (ATFs) including acoustic admittance, acoustic impedance, acoustic pressure reflectance, acoustic energy reflectance, and acoustic energy absorbance.

An ATF for middle ear assessment typically is measured using a sound stimulus (e.g., sinusoid, chirp, click, etc.) presented to an earphone inserted in the ear canal. The sound presented by the earphone is the input and the acoustic response is the output. An ATF can be defined as the ratio of the output response to the acoustic input at each frequency. In the case of admittance measurements, the ATF is defined in terms of the volume velocity

and the sound pressure. The volume velocity is the rate at which the acoustic displacement over a surface varies with time. This may be thought of in terms of a speaker cone in sinusoidal motion and the rate at which air molecules are swept out by the movement of the cone.

The *real* component of admittance, which is in phase with the sound pressure, is called the acoustic conductance, and the *imaginary* component, which is 90 degrees out of phase with the sound pressure, is called the acoustic susceptance. Acoustic impedance is simply the inverse of acoustic admittance. The real component of impedance is the acoustic resistance and the imaginary component is the acoustic reactance.

When a probe is sealed in the external auditory canal for an admittance measurement of middle ear function, the admittance of the volume of air between the probe and the tympanic membrane compromises the measurement so that the admittance of the ear canal and the middle ear admittance are combined when evaluated at the plane of the probe. Tympanometry at low frequencies allows the ear canal admittance magnitude to be subtracted from the total admittance at peak tympanometric pressure to derive the admittance of the middle ear.

Another type of ATF for middle ear measurement is based on the directional path of sound down the ear canal as the incident sound energy is transported from the source (probe) to the tympanic membrane (TM). At the TM some of the sound is absorbed by the middle ear, but some is reflected back along the ear canal, and thus the pressure at the probe microphone is the result of the addition of the incident sound wave and the reflected sound wave. The acoustic pressure reflectance is an ATF which is the ratio of the reflected pressure to the incident pressure at a given frequency, and contains both magnitude and phase information for the incident and reflected pressures. As sound power is proportional to the mean-squared sound pressure, power reflectance (also termed energy reflectance) is the square of the magnitude of the pressure reflectance. This represents the proportion of sound energy reflected by the tympanic membrane. The ATF "absorbance" (one minus energy reflectance) represents the proportion of sound energy absorbed by the middle ear. Because energy is conserved, the incident energy is equal to the sum of the energy reflected at the tympanic membrane and the energy absorbed by the middle ear, assuming that minimal sound energy is absorbed by the ear canal (which generally holds true in adults). Absorbance varies from 1.0 meaning that all the energy was absorbed by the middle ear to 0.0 meaning that all the energy was reflected from the middle ear.

One attractive property of energy reflectance and absorbance is that, unlike admittance, it is relatively independent of the location of measurement in the ear canal. This allows for a direct measure of middle ear function without concern for ear canal effects. However, for low frequencies in infant ears this is only an approximation, as discussed below.

Wideband ATFs may be measured over a wide frequency range similar to the traditional audiogram. Wideband energy reflectance is calculated by first deriving the wideband impedance in the ear canal using a probe for which the Thevenin impedance and pressure response have been determined by prior calibration (Allen, 1986; Keefe, Ling, & Bulen, 1992). The impedance is then compared to the characteristic impedance of the ear canal using standard transformations (Keefe et al., 1992) to derive the pressure reflectance coefficient, R, which is then squared to derive the energy reflectance, $\mathfrak{R}$. Absorbance is then calculated as $1 - \mathfrak{R}$ as a function of frequency.

Figure 7–1 shows the typical energy reflectance at ambient pressure for the left ear of a 30-year-old adult male (S1) with normal hearing. Energy reflectance is near 1.0 around 0.2 kHz showing the inefficiency of the middle ear in the low frequencies. This decreases with increasing frequency from 0.2 kHz to a minimum near 3.0 kHz, and then increases at higher frequencies. S1's absorbance for the same ear at ambient pressure is shown in Figure 7–2. Also shown in this figure is the 5th to 95th percentile and mean of normative data for energy absorbance based on the data of Feeney, Grant, and Marryott (2003a) for 75 ears (20 men and 20 women) of young adults (mean age 21 yr). S1's data fall well within the 5th to 95th percentile of normative data.

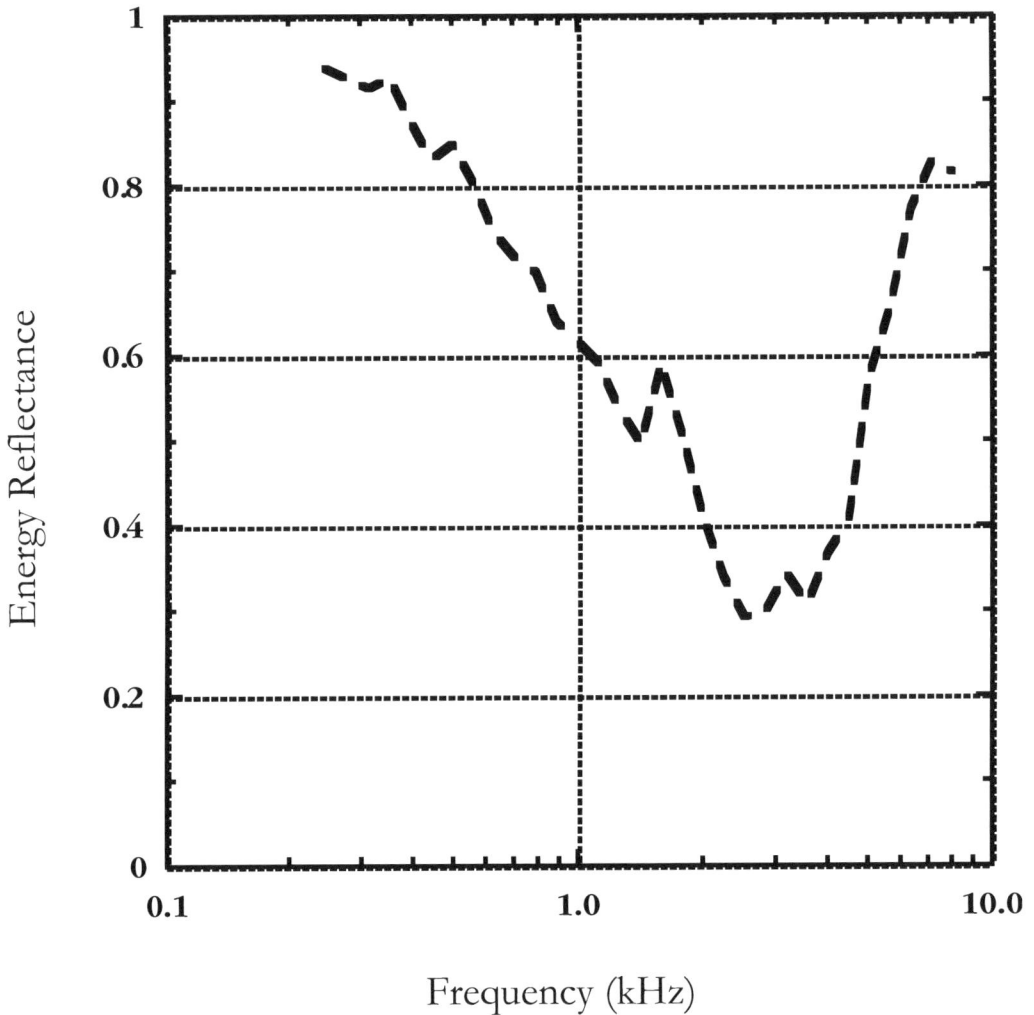

FIGURE 7–1. One-sixth-octave energy reflectance of the left ear of a young adult male (S1) with normal hearing.

ATF ANALYSIS OF MIDDLE EAR FUNCTION IN ADULTS

Normative Data

Mean young-adult third-octave absorbance data from Feeney and Sanford (2004) are shown in Figure 7–3. These are similar to the data of S1 in Figure

7–2. Absorbance is close to 0 at low frequencies, which means that little energy is absorbed by the middle ear in this frequency range. There is a broad maximum of absorbance around 2.0 to 4.0 kHz, and absorbance decreases at higher frequencies up to the frequency limit of 6.0 kHz. The elderly group data in Figure 7–3 show a similar low absorbance at low frequencies as in

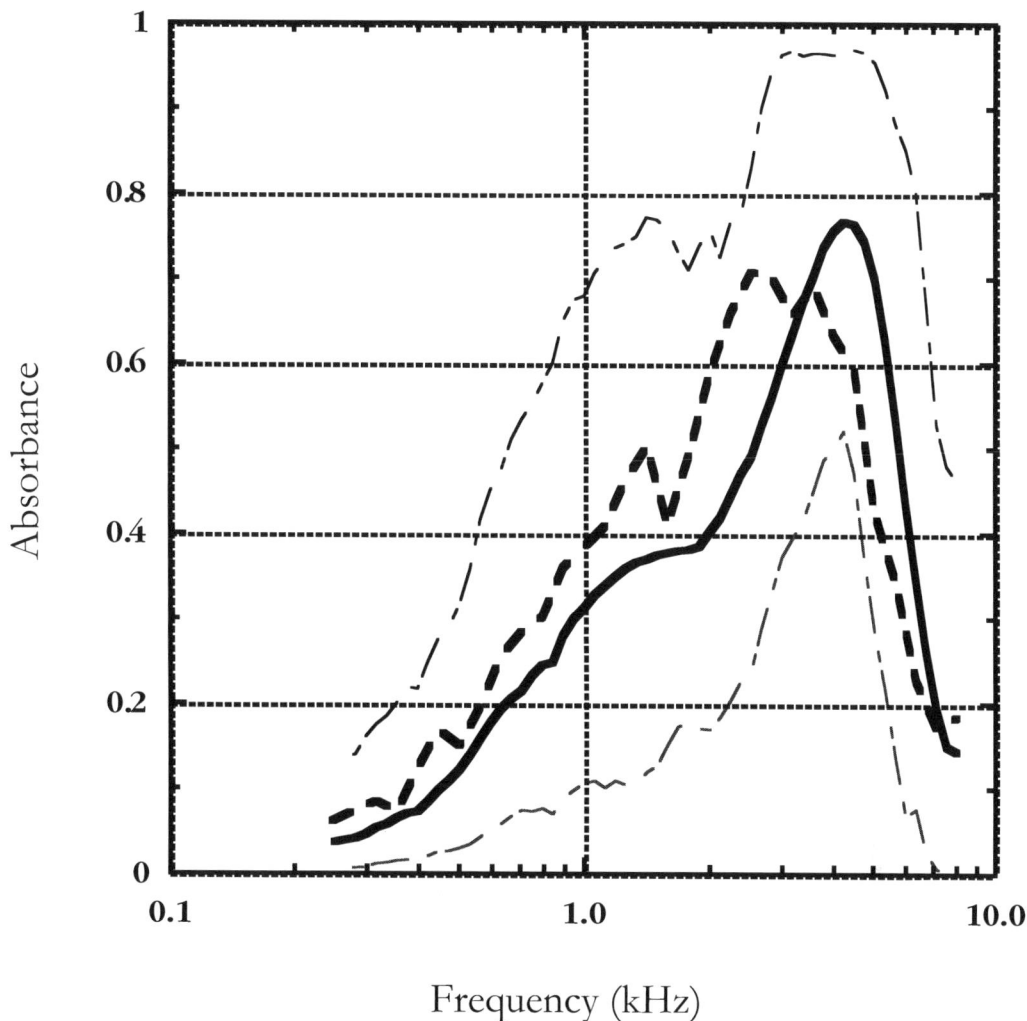

FIGURE 7–2. Absorbance (1–Reflectance) data for the same ear of Subject S1 (*thick dashed line*). Also plotted are the 5th to 95th percentiles of the 1/12th octave normative absorbance data (*thin dashed lines*) for 75 ears of young adults with normal hearing from Feeney et al. (2003a) along with the mean adult absorbance from that study (*thick solid line*).

younger adults, but the patterns diverge between 1.0 and 4.0 kHz. Absorbance was found to be greater in the elderly subjects between 0.8 and 2.0 kHz, but reduced compared to the young adult peak around 5.0 kHz. This was interpreted to suggest that on average the middle ear decreases in stiffness with age, contrary to findings from some previous work (Ruah, Schachern, Zelterman, Paparella, & Yoon, 1991). Significant group gender differences were reported by Feeney and Sanford (2004) with young adult women showing 10% lower mean absorbance at 0.8 and 1.0 kHz than men, but nearly 20% higher

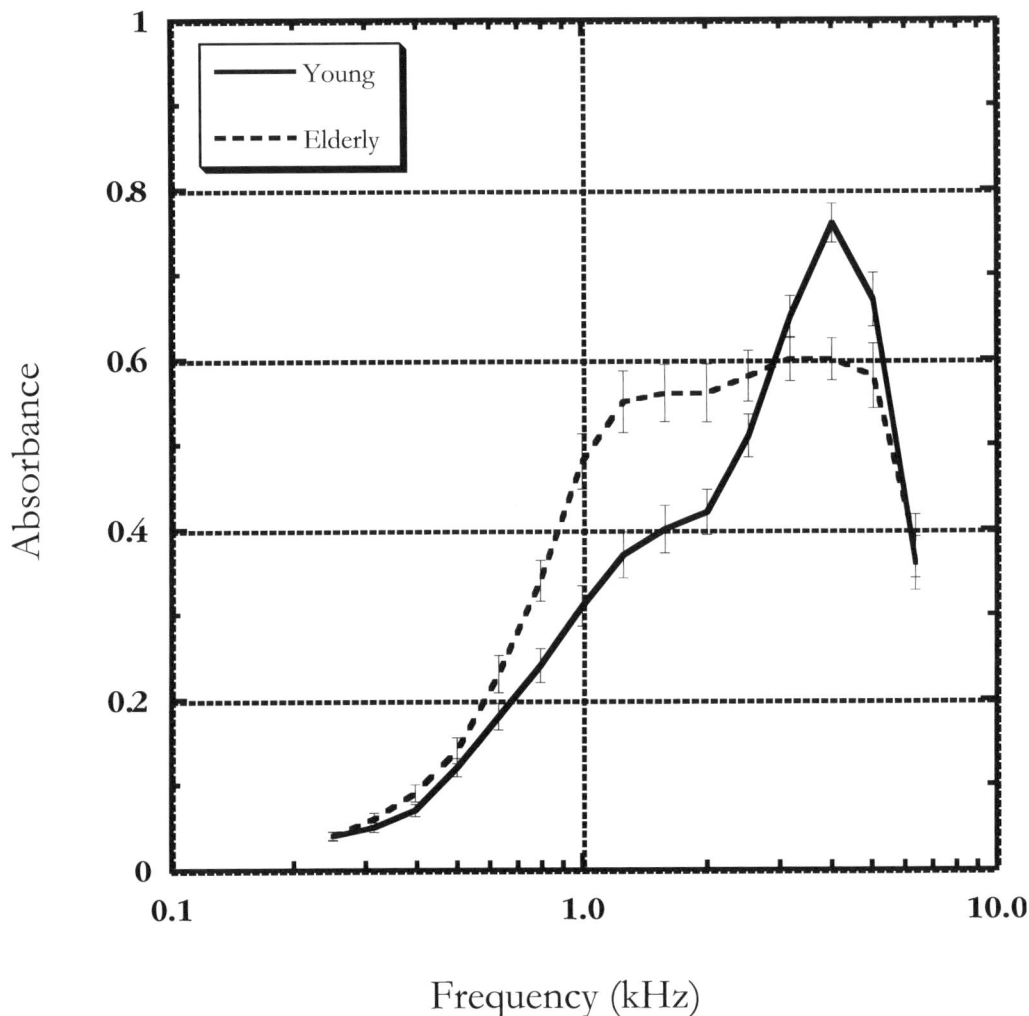

FIGURE 7–3. Third octave mean absorbance at ambient pressure for 40 young (mean age = 21 yr) and 30 older adults (mean age = 71 yr) based on the data of Feeney and Sanford (2004). Error bars represent ±1 standard error.

absorbance at 5.0 kHz. No gender differences were found for the elderly group.

S1's left ear was tested again with wideband absorbance *tympanometry* and the results are shown in Figure 7–4. This three-dimensional plot shows absorbance as a function of pressure and frequency. Wideband energy reflectance tympanometry normative data (0.25 to 11.3 kHz) were first described by Margolis, Saly, and Keefe (1999) in 20 adults with normal hearing. Reflectance was measured at ambient pressure and at a series of ear canal pressures that were manually adjusted. Keefe and Simmons (2003) first reported wideband absorbance at a series of static pressures in 42 ears of normal-hearing adults. As part of a developmental study, Sanford and Feeney (2008) obtained wideband ATFs for adults with normal hearing. They also obtained ATF data during series of static pressure changes to develop wideband tympanograms. Their adult data were in good agreement with the data of Keefe and Simmons (2003) obtained using a similar method. Liu, Sanford, Ellison, Fitzpatrick, Gorga, and Keefe (2008) developed a system for measuring wideband absorbance tympanometry using a pressure sweep in the ear canal (+200 to −300 daPa) for rapid data acquisition by presenting a series of clicks during the pressure sweep. In adult ears with normal hearing, their wideband ATF tympanograms were similar to those obtained using a series of static pressures rather than a pressure sweep (Keefe & Simmons, 2003; Margolis et al., 1999; Sanford & Feeney, 2008). As shown in Figure 7–4 for the normal ear of S1, the wideband absorbance tympanogram obtained using a pressure sweep has a typical "spine" ascending

from low to mid frequencies near ambient pressure. The tympanogram reaches a peak in the 2.0 to 4.0 kHz region before decreasing at higher frequencies.

Wideband ATFs may also be used to measure the acoustic stapedial reflex (ASR). The data in Figure 7–5 show shifts in absorbance as a function of broadband noise activator level for a wideband ipsilateral ASR threshold test on a young adult; the probe signal for this test was a click. Shifts in absorbance were determined by comparing an absorbance response in a baseline condition prior to the activator presentation to the absorbance response immediately after the activator ended. Note that the acoustic reflex induced a decrease in absorbance at frequencies below about 1.0 kHz for the highest three activator levels, along with a small increase in absorbance around 1.5 kHz. There was minimal change in absorbance due to the ASR at frequencies above about 2.0 kHz. The ASR threshold for these data in Figure 7–5 was determined to be

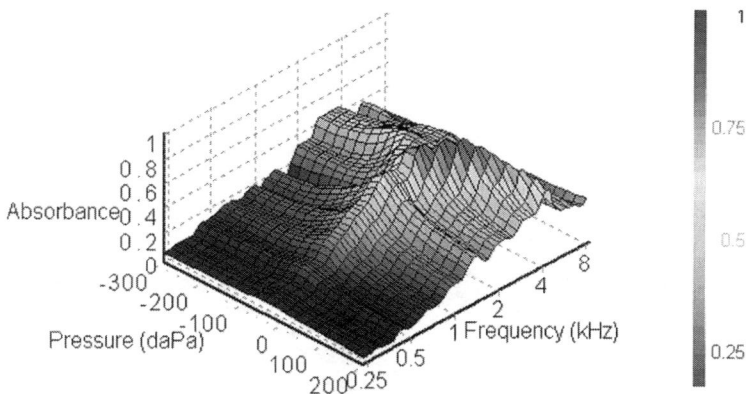

FIGURE 7–4. Wideband absorbance as a function of ear canal pressure from +200 to −300 daPa and frequency from 0.25 to 8.0 kHz for the same adult subject (S1).

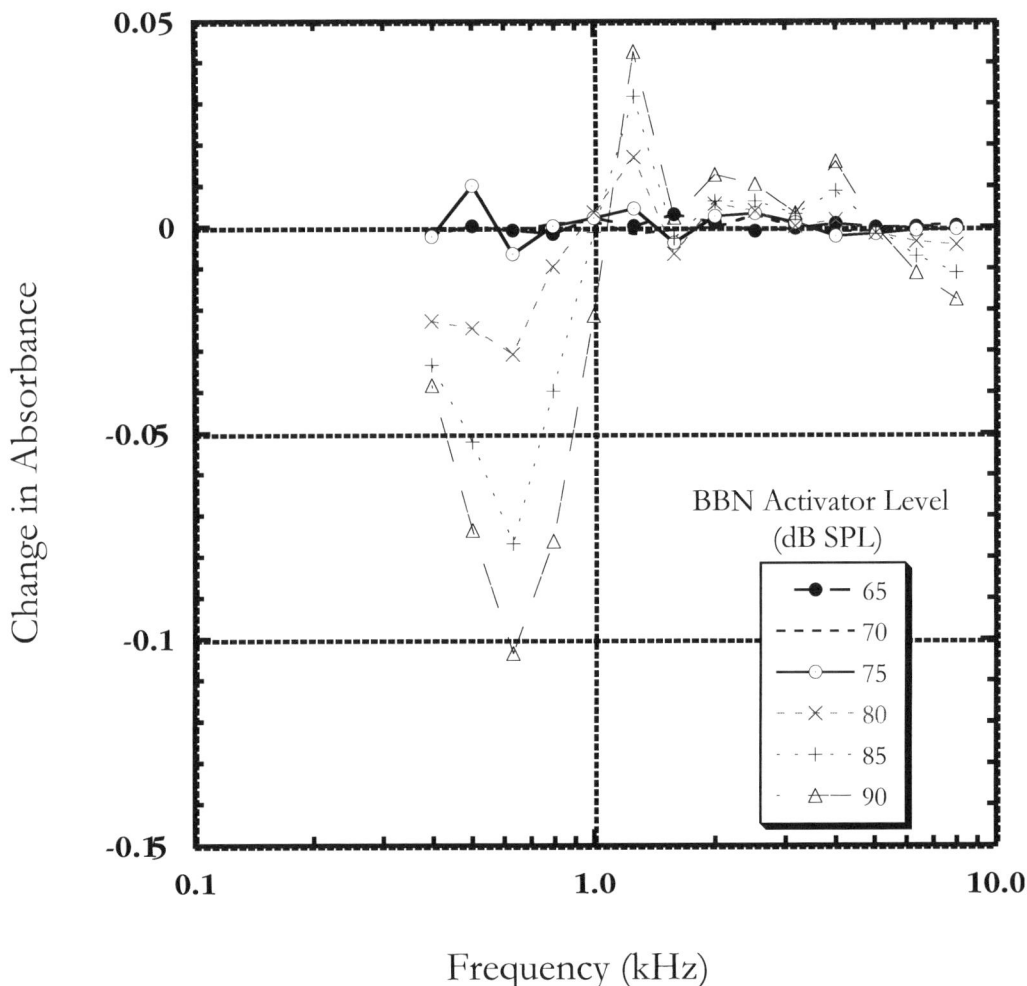

FIGURE 7–5. Shifts in absorbance as a function of frequency during a wideband ATF reflex threshold test for a young adult; the activator stimulus was a broadband noise. A negative shift indicates a decrease in absorbance during the stapedius reflex contraction. The reflex threshold was determined to be 80 dB SPL based on these data.

80 dB SPL based on the magnitude of the shifts and the correlation in shape between successive responses to the various activator levels.

Feeney and Keefe (1999) first measured ASR responses using wideband reflectance, absorbance and admittance ATFs. In that study the probe signal was a wideband chirp that replaced the 0.226-kHz tone, the traditional probe signal. The activator signals were contralateral pure tones. A method to determine ASR thresholds using wideband ATFs was presented by Feeney and Keefe (2001) who developed statistical tests of the wideband shifts in the ATFs. Using this method, Feeney, Keefe, and Marryott (2003b) found that contralateral ASR thresholds averaged 12 dB lower than clinical thresholds for the same tonal activators. Therefore, the use of wideband ATFs may provide a more sensitive measure of ASR threshold. However, Schairer, Ellison, Fitzpatrick, and Keefe (2007) found only a few dB reduction in *ipsilateral* ASR thresholds using wideband ATFs.

Application of ATFs to the Evaluation of Middle Ear Disorders and Conductive Hearing Loss

Wideband ATFs at ambient pressure have been used in several studies of patients with middle ear disorders. Feeney et al. (2003a) presented several cases in which wideband reflectance ATFs at ambient pressure were obtained in ears with otoscelerosis, ossicular discontinuity, otitis media, and perforation of the tympanic membrane. There was a very different pattern of wideband energy reflectance in ears with otosclerosis compared to ossicular disarticulation. Ears with otosclerosis had energy reflectance greater than the 95th percentile of the normative data at frequencies below 1.0 kHz, whereas ears with ossicular discontinuity had a deep notch in energy reflectance at around 0.7 kHz. Ears with serous otitis media had energy reflectance near 1.0 for most of the frequency range, whereas subjects with tympanic membrane perforation had energy reflectance near 0.0 at frequencies below 1.0 kHz. Allen, Jeng, and Levitt (2005) reported similar results for several cases of otitis media and otosclerosis.

Group data on 28 ears of patients with otosclerosis were compared with data from 62 ears from normal-hearing adults by Shahnaz, Bork, Polka, Longridge, Bell, and Westerberg (2009). They compared 0.226-kHz tympanometry, multifrequency tympanometry, and wideband energy reflectance in these subjects. Multifrequency tympanometry was used to calculate the frequency at which the susceptance and conductance components of admittance were at a phase angle of 45 degrees (F45°), which has been shown to be a sensitive predictor of ossicular fixation (Shahnaz & Polka, 1997, 2002). Shahnaz et al. (2009) found that patients with otosclerosis had higher energy reflectance than controls at frequencies between 0.4 and 1.0 kHz, which is consistent with the data from Feeney et al. (2003a). Shahnaz et al. (2009) also found that energy reflectance at 0.5 kHz did a good job of distinguishing otosclerotic from normal ears with an area under the receiver operating characteristic (ROC) curve of 0.86 compared to 0.50 for static acoustic admittance as obtained using traditional 0.226 kHz tympanometry. F45° was essentially as successful as energy reflectance at 0.5 kHz with an area under the ROC curve of 0.84. Shahnaz et al. (2009) suggested that F45° might be combined with energy reflectance to improve test performance.

Feeney, Grant, and Mills (2009) conducted a human cadaver temporal-bone study to evaluate the source of the low-frequency notch in energy reflectance that had been reported for ears with ossicular discontinuity by Feeney et al. (2003a). Energy reflectance was measured at ambient pressure in three conditions: a baseline condition with the ossicular chain intact; a second condition with the ossicular chain severed at the incudostapedial joint; and finally with the defect repaired with dental cement. The characteristic low-frequency notch in energy reflectance at around 0.7 kHz was observed in each of a series of five temporal bones. The results showed that the notch in energy reflectance at 0.7 kHz occurred at the new resonance frequency of the middle ear when corrected for ear canal admittance. This energy reflectance pattern may be useful in distinguishing ossicular discontinuity from otosclerosis.

Wideband reflectance measurements at ambient pressure were also used by Piskorski, Keefe, Simmons, and Gorga (1999) to predict the presence of conductive hearing loss in children at risk for otitis media with effusion. Using a clinical decision theory approach, they reported that for a fixed sensitivity of 0.80, the ATF predictor had a specificity of 0.93 compared to a specificity of 0.70 for the best predictor based on 0.226-kHz tympanometry. These results show the advantage of using a wideband ATF measure over traditional 0.226-kHz tympanometry in detecting conductive hearing loss in an at-risk population.

Keefe and Simmons (2003) used wideband absorbance tympanometry in adults and older children to predict the presence of conductive hearing loss in 42 normal ears and 18 ears with conductive hearing loss. They used a clinical decision theory approach to compare the use of three different measures to predict conductive hearing loss: static acoustic admittance at 0.226- kHz, absorbance at ambient pressure, and absorbance tympanometry. For a fixed specificity of 0.90 the sensitivity was 0.94 for absorbance tympanometry, 0.72 for ambient-pressure absorbance, and 0.28 for static acoustic admittance at 0.226 kHz. For predicting conductive hearing loss, wideband power-based ATFs may be a more sensitive tool than traditional tympanometry in adults and older children.

DEVELOPMENTAL STUDIES IN WIDEBAND ATFS

Understanding maturational changes in the infant middle ear and their effects on transfer of sound energy through the middle ear is important for our understanding of developmental processes in the auditory system and for the development of clinical norms for hearing and middle ear assessment. Maturational changes in the middle ear may also impact the interpretation of auditory brainstem response (ABR) tests and to a greater extent, otoacoustic emission (OAE) measurements, which depend on both forward and reverse transfer of sound energy through the middle ear. The studies reviewed in the following section highlight the effects of infant middle ear maturation on ear canal-based ATF measurements.

ATFs: Ambient Pressure Conditions

Keefe, Bulen, Arehart, and Burns (1993) first described maturational effects for ATF measurements obtained at ambient ear canal pressure for 1-, 3-, 6-, 12-, and 24-month-old infants and children and for a group of adults. Figure 7–6 shows averaged absorbance for the subjects in the Keefe et al. (1993) study and for a group of neonates from Keefe, Folsom, Gorga, Vohr, Bulen, and Norton (2000). The thickest dark line represents adult data, which, for the most part has the lowest absorbance of any age group. This figure shows that as age decreases absorbance generally increases. Keefe et al. (1993) identified significant dif-

ferences in absorbance between infant groups, with most differences observed between 0.5 and 6.0 kHz. Although changes in absorbance with age occurred across a wide frequency range (0.125 to 10.0 kHz), the greatest changes occurred below 1.0 kHz. Figure 7–6 shows that absorbance data for neonates are close to 0.8 at 0.25 kHz, but approach 0 for ages 6 months and greater. The higher degree of absorbance below 1.0 kHz for neonates and young infants may not translate into

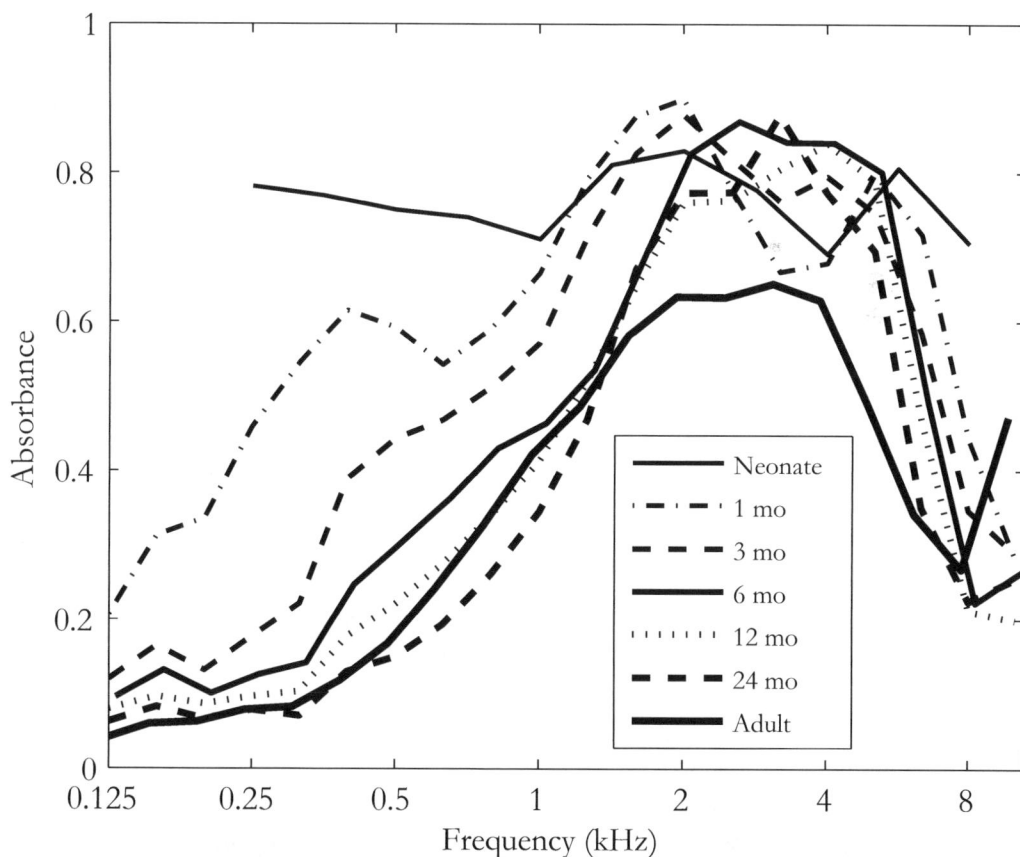

FIGURE 7–6. ATF absorbance data from Keefe et al. 1993 (infants and adults) and Keefe et al. 2000 (neonates). Figure from "Physiological mechanisms assessed by aural acoustic transfer functions" by M. P. Feeney and D. H. Keefe in *Translational Perspectives in Auditory Neuroscience* by K. Tremblay and R. Burkard (Eds.) (in press). Copyright © Plural Publishing, Inc. All rights reserved. Used with permission.

more sound energy being transferred to the inner ear, but may be explained by a more absorbent infant ear canal shunting lower frequency energy away from the middle ear (Keefe et al., 1993). Consistent with findings in previous work utilizing multifrequency tympanometry (Holte, Margolis, & Cavanaugh, 1991), changes in ATF responses for higher frequencies may be due to maturational shifts from a mass dominated to stiffness dominated middle ear system.

Sanford and Feeney (2008) reported ambient ATF data for 4-, 12-, and 24-week-old infants and adults (20 participants in each age group). The bottom panel of Figure 7–7 shows adult absorbance data from that study, as well as adult data from Keefe et al. (1993), and Feeney et al. (2003a) with a similar absorbance pattern across studies. Infant data (upper 3 panels of Figure 7–7) from Sanford and Feeney (2008) and Keefe et al. (1993) are similar for each age group. The most dramatic changes in absorbance for infants occur between 4 and 12 weeks of age as low frequency absorbance decreases, becoming more adultlike, and an absorbance minimum between 3.0 and 5.0 kHz becomes less pronounced with increasing age.

Shahnaz (2008) obtained ATF data from 26 infants (49 ears) in a neonatal intensive care unit (NICU). These infants had an average gestational age of 37.8 weeks and ranged in age from 32 to 51 weeks. ATF results (reflectance) were similar to data from 4-week-old infants shown in Figure 7–7 (top panel) with an absorbance minimum occurring around 4.0 kHz, rising to a peak near 6.0 kHz, then descending as frequency increased.

More recent work by Werner, Levi, and Keefe (2010) reported ambient ATF measurement data for 458 infants from 2 to 9 months and 210 adults. Figure 7–8 shows data arranged by age for participants 2 to 3 months, 5 to 9 months, and adults. Werner et al. (2010) reported significant differences in absorbance across age, with most differences occurring between 0.75 and 4.0 kHz. These data and the data of Figure 7–7 show a similar developmental trend of decreasing absorbance, especially below about 3.0 kHz, as a function of increasing age from infancy to young adulthood.

Ambient ATF data from 97 infants and children ranging in age from 3 days to 47 months were presented by Hunter, Tubaugh, Jackson, and Propes (2008). Contrary to previous studies, they did not find significant age-related differences in ATF measurements across frequency, with the exception of 6.0 kHz. Hunter et al. (2008) suggested that differences in probe design and calibration methods could account for the differences observed in their study, relative to previous work. In addition, Hunter et al. (2008) used less discrete age ranges than previous work (e.g., 3 days to 2 months, 12 to 23 months, etc.), which may have obscured significant maturational differences in ATF measurements observed in earlier studies.

ATFs: Tympanometric (Ear Canal Pressure) Conditions

Although the reasons for differences in immittance characteristics between adults and infants are not fully known, it has

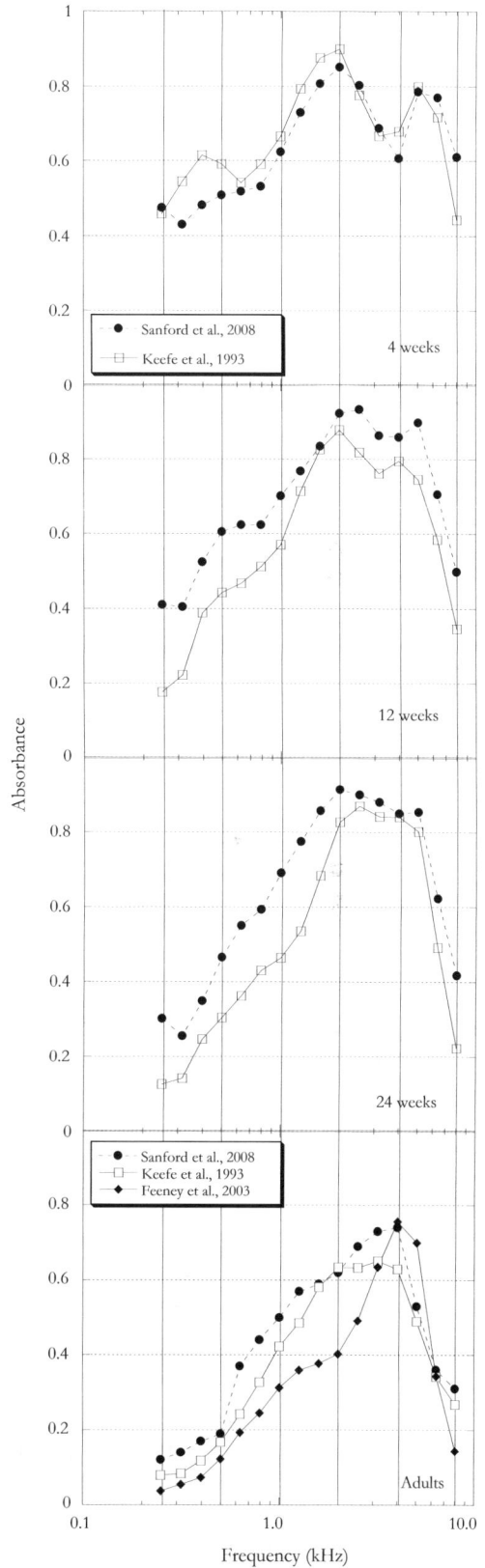

FIGURE 7–7. Group mean one-third-octave ambient energy absorbance as a function of frequency for adults and infants at 4, 12, and 24 weeks of age from Sanford and Feeney (2008); $N = 20$ ears for each age group. Comparison data at each age are from work by Keefe et al. (1993). The numbers of subjects for each age group in Keefe et al. (1993) are 15 one-month-old, 18 3-month-old, and 11 6-month-old infants, and 10 adults. The bottom panel also includes absorbance data from 75 ears of young adults from Feeney et al. (2003a).

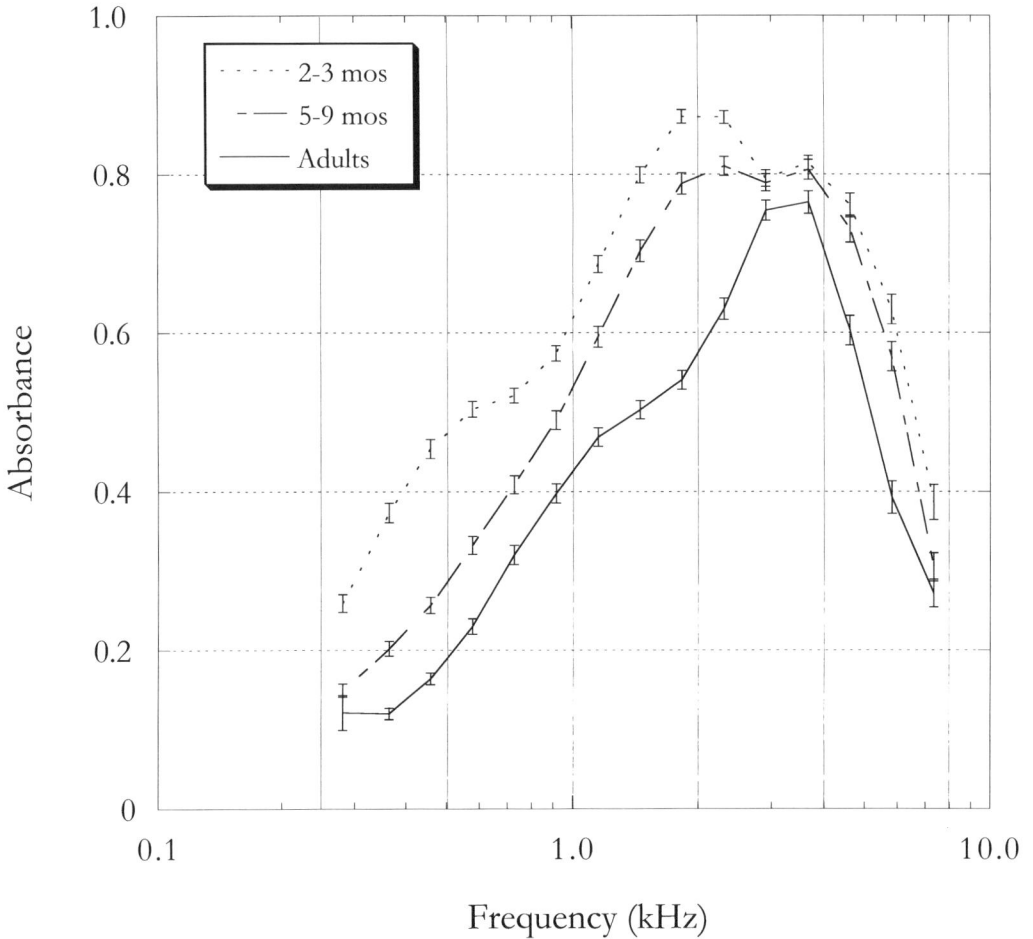

FIGURE 7–8. Mean ear canal energy absorbance as a function of frequency from Werner et al. (2010) for 2 to 3 and 5 to 9-month-old infants and a group of adults. Error bars represent ± 1 standard error of the mean (SEM).

been shown that developmental changes in the infant external and middle ear contribute to differences in acoustic measures of middle ear function (Holte et al., 1991; Keefe et al., 1993; Meyer, Jardine, & Deverson, 1997). Although the effects of ear canal pressure on admittance and ATF measurements in adults is fairly well understood (Margolis et al., 1999), there is less understand-

ing regarding the effects of introducing ear canal pressure in newborn and young infant ears.

To investigate the hypothesis that pressure-induced changes in the external ear canal influence immittance measurements, Holte, Cavanaugh, and Margolis (1990) introduced positive and negative pressure pulses in the ear canal and used video-monitoring to determine a percent change in ear canal diameter relative to resting diameter. This was found to decrease as a function of age, dropping from an average 18% change (as great as 70% change in some infants) at 1 to 7 days to no change at 4 months of age. Holte and colleagues reported that in some cases, where no ear canal wall motion was observed, there were still multiple peaks in the 0.226-kHz tympanograms. Correlations that were computed to assess the relationship between complexity of tympanometric patterns and amount of wall distention failed to reach significance. Based on this result, the authors suggested that ear canal wall mobility and tympanometric patterns were not related. The general trends observed by Holte et al. (1990) suggest using acoustic ear canal measurements at multiple frequencies to more accurately assess an infant's middle ear status.

Just as the addition of ear canal pressure changes have increased the usefulness of low-frequency admittance measurements in adults and children, it has been hypothesized that wideband ATF measurements may reveal more developmental effects and be more diagnostically useful if they are obtained in the presence of ear canal pressure changes (Keefe & Simmons, 2003; Margolis et al., 1999; Piskorski et al., 1999). Sanford and Feeney (2008) obtained ATF measurements at varying static ear canal pressures in 4-, 12-, and 24-week-old infants and young adults. Results showed developmental changes in wideband ATF measurements that varied as a function of frequency (Figure 7–9).

Absorbance measurements in infants at frequencies from 0.25 to 0.75 kHz showed as much as a 30% change in mean absorbance with changes in static ear canal pressure from +200 to −200 daPa. The effects of ear canal pressure resulted in minimal developmental differences in absorbance at frequencies from 0.75 to 2.0 kHz, suggestive of a developmentally stable frequency range. At high frequencies from 2.0 to 6.0 kHz negative pressures caused decreased absorbance and positive pressures caused increased absorbance in the 4-week-old infants. This high-frequency effect was not observed for older infants. Although a specific time line of infant ear canal development has not been fully described, some of the age-related effects of pressure observed in ATF responses may be the result of more compliant ear canal walls (i.e., more susceptible to collapse) or less rigid coupling of the ossicles (Saunders, Kaltenback, & Relkin, 1983), which become more resistant to changes in pressure with age.

ATFs: Stapedial Reflex Test

A number of studies have revealed effects of middle ear development on the measurement of the ASR. For example, when low-frequency probe tones (0.22/0.226 kHz) have been used to measure the reflex in newborns, approximately 90% of healthy infants have absent reflexes (Abahazi & Greenberg, 1977; Bennett, 1975; Jerger, Jerger, Mauldin, & Segal, 1974; Keith, 1973;

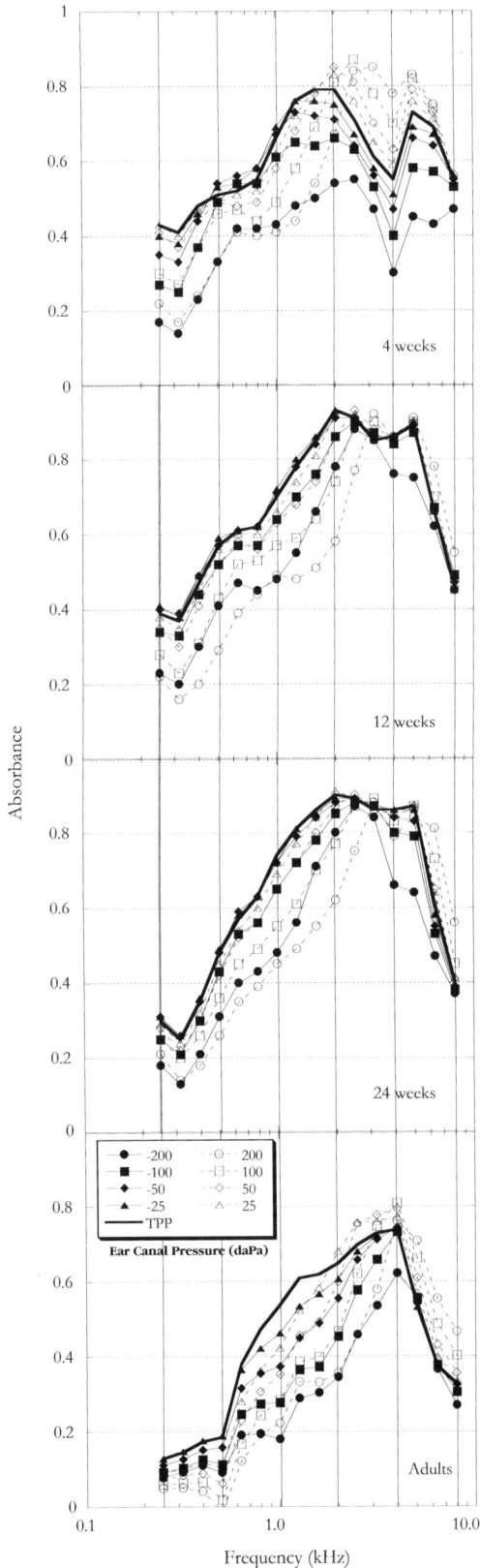

FIGURE 7–9. Group mean one-third-octave energy absorbance plotted as a function of ear canal-pressure conditions and frequency for 4-, 12-, and 24-week-old infants and adults from Sanford and Feeney (2008); $N = 20$ for each group. Filled symbols represent negative ear canal pressure conditions and open symbols represent positive ear canal pressure conditions.

Weatherby & Bennett, 1980). However, Weatherby and Bennett (1980), using a variable-frequency impedance device, reported that 100% of newborns had measurable reflexes for probe frequencies from 0.8 to 1.8 kHz, when they had been absent using a 0.22-kHz probe tone. Moreover, reflex thresholds in these infants were found to decrease by 10 dB with increasing probe frequency, showing that reflex threshold sensitivity changes with the probe frequency independent of the activator stimulus used to evoke the reflex. Therefore, using a single-probe frequency to measure reflex thresholds for all ages could result in a distorted view of reflex threshold development.

Feeney and Sanford (2005) examined changes in ATFs induced by the contralateral acoustic stapedial reflex in five 6-week-old infants and in one young adult using wideband shifts in admittance and energy reflectance ATFs. The probe signal used to monitor acoustic changes in the ear canal consisted of 40-ms electrical chirps with a bandwidth from 0.2 to 10.0 kHz. The reflex activator presented to the contralateral ear was a band-pass noise from 0.25 to 11.0 kHz presented at a maximum overall level of 90 dB SPL measured in the ear canal. Reflex-induced ATF shifts were then obtained by subtracting measurements obtained during a quiet baseline from those obtained in the presence of a contralateral activator noise. Reflexes were detected by calculating a cross-correlation between one-twelfth-octave ATF measurements for the highest activator level and responses to lower levels. The reflex-induced shifts

in ATFs for the infant ears were similar in pattern to adult responses, but were shifted higher in frequency by around 0.5 kHz. Infant reflexes were more successfully detected when the cross-correlation was calculated from 1.0 to 8.0 kHz, whereas adult reflexes were more successfully detected for a cross-correlation from 0.25 to 2.0 kHz. This wideband acoustic reflex method may be useful in capturing the most robust frequency region for acoustic reflex detection across postnatal middle ear development.

ATF ANALYSIS OF MIDDLE EAR FUNCTION FOR NEWBORN HEARING SCREENING AND INFANT MIDDLE EAR DISORDERS

Current Newborn Hearing Screening (NHS) guidelines published by the Joint Committee on Infant Hearing (JCIH) endorse hearing screening, as well as timely and appropriate follow-up and intervention through the establishment and development of early hearing detection and intervention (EHDI) programs (JCIH, 2007). The initial goal of an EHDI program is to correctly classify an infant's hearing status so that timely and appropriate intervention can take place as needed.

Auditory brainstem response (ABR) and otoacoustic emission (OAE) tests are the primary NHS tests to determine hearing status. It has been recommended that an infant who does not pass one or both of these birth-admission screening tests be referred for follow-up re-screening tests. It has been suggested that a significant number of infants who are referred for follow-up testing do so as a result of congenital, middle ear dysfunction most likely caused by conditions such as vernix occluding the ear canal, middle ear effusion, residual amniotic fluid or mesenchyme in the middle ear space (Chang, Vohr, Norton, & Lekas, 1993; Doyle, Burggraaff, Fujikawa, & Kim, 1997; Kok, van Zanten, & Brocaar, 1992; Rosenfeld et al., 2004; Takahara, Sando, Hashida, & Shibahara, 1986). Because both ABR and OAE test results are influenced by ear canal and middle ear factors, confirmation of hearing status is not complete until effects of middle ear dysfunction are ruled out. Although thought to be mostly transient in nature, research suggests that middle ear dysfunction can persist during the first few months of life and beyond (Boone, Bower, & Martin, 2005; Doyle, Kong, Strobel, Dallaire, & Ray, 2004).

Because the outpatient follow-up re-screening phase is a critical time where decisions regarding follow-up and intervention are made, minimizing delays in classification of cochlear and middle ear status is important. Furthermore, the goals endorsed for follow-up testing include outpatient re-screening by 1 month of age and if needed, medical and audiologic assessment completed no later than 3 months of age (JCIH, 2007). Therefore, a valid, objective test of middle ear status would assist clinicians and health care providers in meeting these goals and provide help with interpretation of screening and diagnostic tests and clinical care decisions.

Because ATF responses provide information about middle ear function in young infants, their usefulness has been evaluated in relation to NHS programs. For example, Keefe, Zhao, Neely, Gorga, and Vohr (2003a) analyzed a subset of data obtained from a two-stage hearing screening protocol (e.g., OAE followed by ABR) that produced a 5% false-positive rate (Keefe et al., 2000). Keefe et al. (2003a) reported significant correlations between two ATF factors and TEOAE responses, suggesting that ATF measures could be useful in interpreting TEOAE responses. Applying ATF factors identified in Keefe et al. (2003a) to a predictive test of middle ear dysfunction on the same subset of infant data, Keefe, Gorga, Neely, Zhao, and Vohr (2003b) showed that the ATF test suggested that middle ear dysfunction was present in 4 out of 5 false-positive results.

Vander Werff, Prieve, and Georgantas (2007) investigated test-retest variability and differences in ambient wideband reflectance measures between a group of infants receiving outpatient hearing screenings with a mean age of 7.6 weeks (SD = 5.3) and another group receiving outpatient diagnostic hearing assessments with a mean age of 12.4 weeks (SD = 8.5). Test-retest variability was lowest for the diagnostic group, on whom testing was performed in a sound-treated booth. The lower test-retest variability in the diagnostic group was attributed to decreased environmental noise. Vander Werff et al. (2007) also reported that infants who failed the

OAE screening had significantly higher reflectance than infants who passed at frequencies from 0.63 to 2.0 kHz, suggesting the potential usefulness of an ATF test in NHS follow-up settings.

Sanford, Keefe, Liu, Fitzpatrick, McCreery, Lewis, and Gorga (2009) evaluated test performance of ATF measurements and 1.0-kHz tympanometry in relation to outcomes on a DPOAE-based NHS test. Distortion-product otoacoustic emission (DPOAE) testing was used to determine the newborn hearing screening status of 455 infant ears (375 passed and 80 referred). Figure 7–10 shows absorbance ATF tympanometry data (50th percentile) for ears that passed the DPOAE test (top panel) and ears that referred (bottom panel). Lower overall absorbance in the refer group is suggestive of a reduction in middle ear efficiency for this group. Clinical decision theory analysis was used to determine the test performance of ATF and 1.0-kHz tests in terms of their ability to classify ears that passed or were referred. The highest area under the ROC curve was 0.87 for an ambient ATF test compared to 0.75 for 1.0 kHz tympanometry. Figure 7–11 shows median ambient-pressure absorbance data for both DPOAE pass and refer ears (solid and dashed lines, respectively) with shaded regions representing the 25th and 75th percentiles for each group. For the most part, ears that passed the DPOAE test had higher absorbance compared to ears that were referred, indicating the importance of middle ear status for interpreting DPOAE test data in newborns.

Similar to Sanford et al. (2009), Hunter, Feeney, Lapsley Miller, Jeng, and Bohning (2010) obtained ATF and 1.0-kHz tympanometry data from a large number of well-baby infants ($N = 324$) undergoing their newborn hearing screening DPOAE test. Hunter et al. (2010) reported that ATF data (plotted in terms of absorbance in Figure 7–12) for infants who were referred on their DPOAE screening were significantly lower than for infants who passed their DPOAE screening for frequencies ranging from 1.0 to 6.0 kHz (Figure 7–12). Using the DPOAE screening outcome as the "gold standard," test performance of ATF and 1.0-kHz tympanometry were assessed in terms of their ability to predict DPOAE outcomes. The three tests evaluated in the ROC analysis included, 1.0-kHz tympanometric data (0.6 mmho used as the cutoff for normal), reflectance at 1.0 kHz, and reflectance at 2.0 kHz. The authors reported that discrete reflectance frequencies of 1.0 and 2.0 kHz were used for the following reasons: (1) for direct comparison to 1.0-kHz tympanometry results (1.0 kHz reflectance) and (2) because 2.0 kHz was the frequency at which the best discrimination between a DPOAE pass and refer was found. Resulting areas under the ROC curve were 0.72 for 1.0-kHz admittance, 0.82 for 1.0-kHz reflectance and 0.90 for 2.0 kHz reflectance, very similar to the ROC results reported by Sanford et al. (2009). These results suggest that ATF measurements may be a useful test to help identify conductive dysfunction during the newborn period.

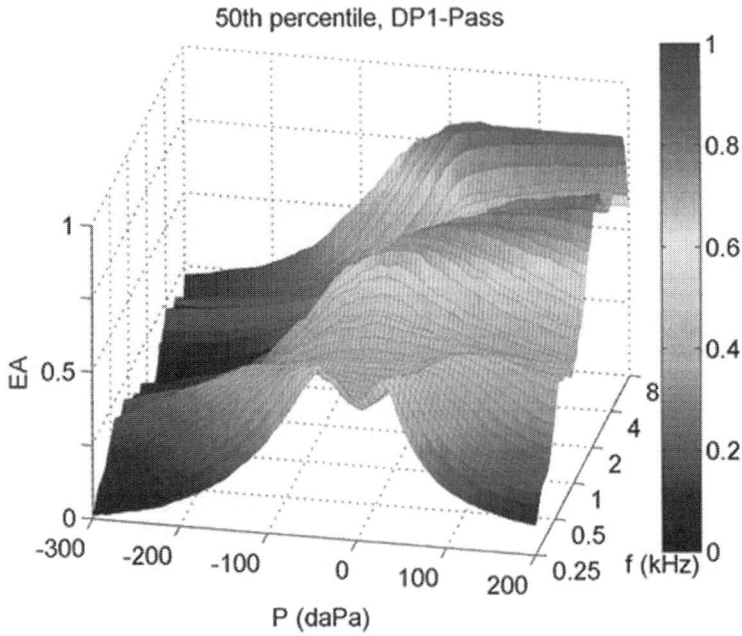

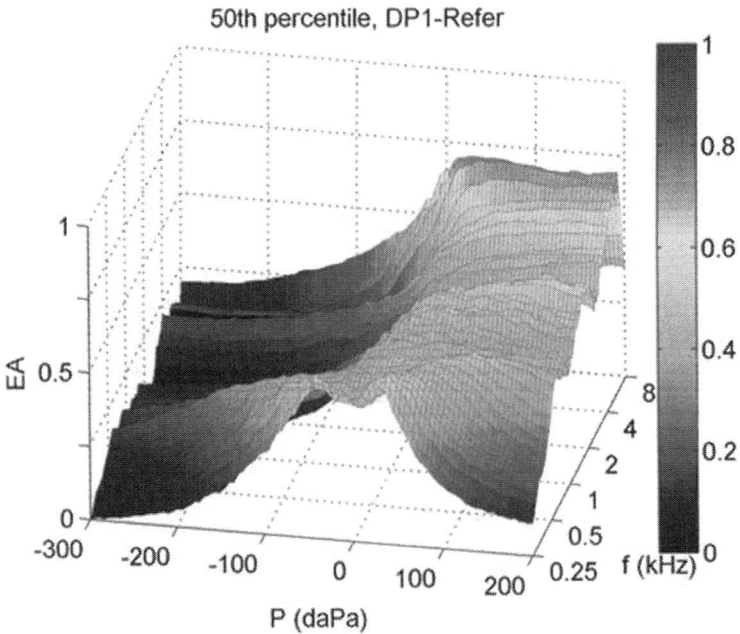

FIGURE 7–10. Group median tympanometric energy absorbance responses from newborn ears for both DPOAE pass and refer groups (*top and bottom*, respectively). The 50th percentile from each group is plotted as energy absorbance (EA) as a joint function of ear canal pressure (*P*) and frequency (*f*). Figure from "Sound-conduction effects on distortion-product otoacoustic emission screening outcomes in newborn infants: Test performance of wideband acoustic transfer functions and 1-kHz tympanometry" by C. A. Sanford, et al. (2009). *Ear and Hearing, 30*(6), 642. Copyright © Lippincott Williams & Wilkins. All rights reserved. Used with permission.

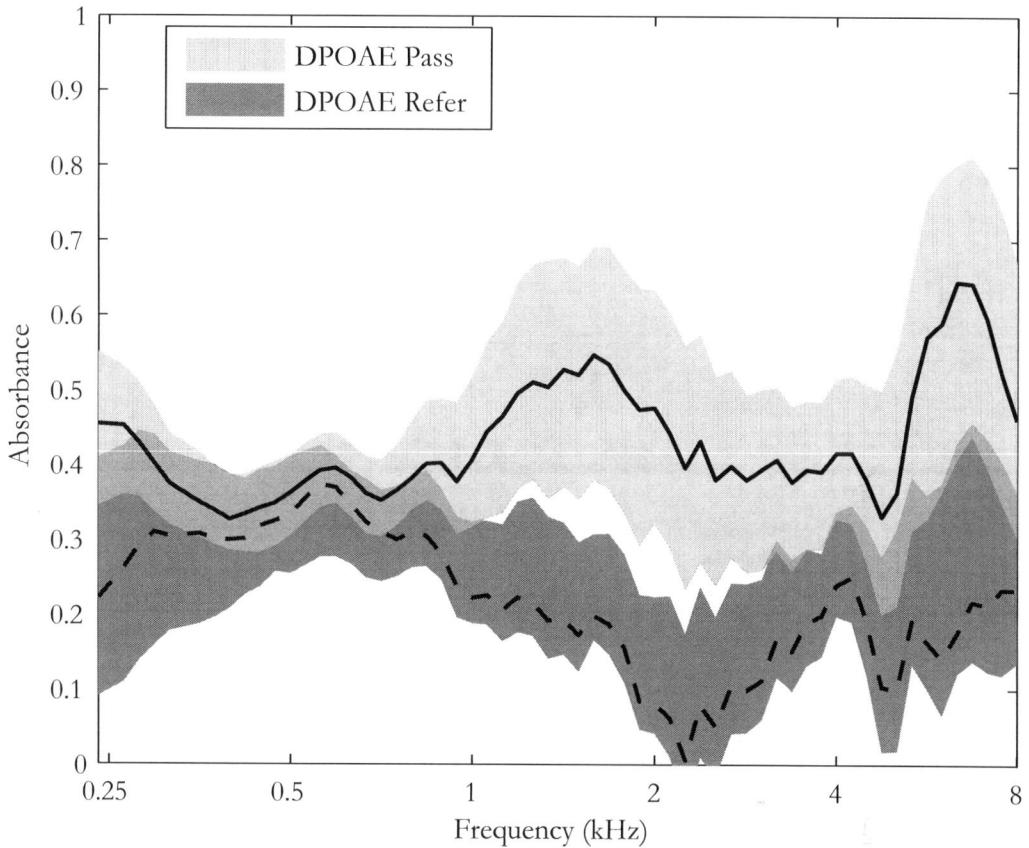

FIGURE 7–11. Group averaged ambient energy absorbance from newborn ears for both DPOAE pass and refer groups from Sanford et al. (2009). Shaded areas denote the 25th to 75th percentile range with *pass* = light gray shading and *refer* = dark gray shading; where there is overlap between the two groups, the dark gray shading can been seen "behind" the light gray shading. Black lines, solid and dashed, represent the 50th percentile for the DPOAE pass and refer groups, respectively. Figure from "Physiological mechanisms assessed by aural acoustic transfer functions" by M. P. Feeney and D. H. Keefe in *Translational Perspectives in Auditory Neuroscience* by K. Tremblay and R. Burkard (Eds.) (in press). Copyright © Plural Publishing, Inc. All rights reserved. Used with permission.

ATFs: Acoustic Stapedial Reflex Test

Keefe, Fitzpatrick, Liu, Sanford, and Gorga (2010) hypothesized that a wideband ATF test battery including wideband ASR thresholds and an ambient ATF test would be more accurate than 1.0-kHz tympanometry in classifying ears that passed or referred on an otoacoustic emission test. Ambient ATF and ipsilateral reflex measurements were gathered from adults, children 3 to 10 years of age, and newborn (well-baby) infants (same infant participants as noted in the discussion of Sanford et al.,

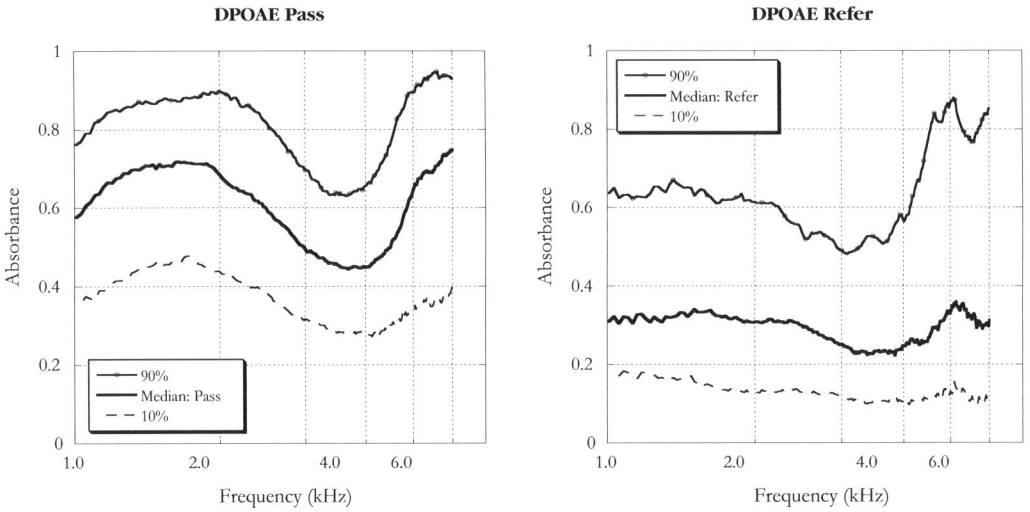

FIGURE 7–12. Absorbance data (median, 10th and 90th percentiles) from newborn ears for both DPOAE pass and refer groups (reflectance data from Hunter et al. [2010] re-plotted in terms of absorbance).

2009). Reflex activator stimuli consisted of broadband-noise activator pulses alternating with click stimuli which served as the wideband ATF probe. The reflex-induced shift in middle ear function was defined as the difference in wideband ATF between the initial pre-activator click response and the final postactivator click response. ASR shifts were calculated separately for the low-frequency region from 0.8 to 2.8 kHz (ASRT-L) and the high-frequency region from 2.8 to 8.0 kHz (ASRT-H). Clinical decision theory analyses were performed to investigate the test performance of 1.0-kHz and ATF tests at classifying newborn hearing screening status. Comparing ASR-H and ASR-L revealed that ASR-L was a more accurate test. A test battery approach, combining an ambient ATF test and ASR-L showed improved test performance over the ATF alone, but the increase in test performance was not significantly different. ASRTs were measured in 97% and 90% of infants who passed or referred on their OAE screening, respectively, using at least one of the ASR-H or ASR-L criteria. It was interesting to note that, although many infants who referred on the screening test still had a measureable ASRT, the median ASRT measured using ASR-L was 24 dB higher in the refer group. Although the presence or absence of an ART was not a good predictor of an OAE pass or refer, the higher ASRTs in the refer group suggest a decrease in middle ear efficiency. Overall, an optimal combination of wideband ATF and ASRT tests performed better than either reflex test alone in predicting OAE screening outcomes, and either ATF test performed better than 1.0-kHz tympanometry.

SUMMARY

Confident application of traditional immittance measurements in young infants has been questioned based on inconsistent test results in the literature. While it is clear that developmental factors in ear canaland/or middle ear characteristics influence immittance results, there still are questions regarding specific relationships between acoustic measures and individual physical characteristics of the young infant ear. A valid neonatal test of middle ear function would be beneficial in interpreting OAE and ABR screening results, and would help improve the management and follow-up care of infants. Additionally, due to the use of untrained screening personnel in many settings, an objective middle ear test that does not rely on subjective interpretation would have usefulness in NHS programs. For example, JCIH (2007, p. 903) states, "Screening technologies that incorporate automated-response detection are necessary to eliminate the need for individual test interpretation, to reduce the effects of screener bias or operator error on test outcome, and to ensure test consistency across infants, test conditions, and screening personnel." Although technologies fitting these criteria currently exist for OAE and ABR testing, a valid, objective test of middle ear function in infants is currently lacking. However, ATF tests and other aural acoustic tests of middle ear function discussed in this book are showing promising results. Because successful conduction of sound into the inner ear relies on middle ear mechanisms, these questions not only apply to measures of middle ear function, but also to investigations of auditory sensitivity. Wideband ATFs provide a view of the acoustic response properties of the middle ear across the critical speech-frequency range, and appear to be good indicators of infant middle ear status.

CASE STUDY

The following case study was chosen to illustrate specific developmental features that are consistent with or diverge from group averaged ATF data. Specifically, similarities and differences between a single subject's longitudinal ATF data and group mean ATF data for infants ranging in age from 1 to 6 months of age are presented. Longitudinal data were obtained from one female infant (S2) who presented with a normal birth history and passed a newborn hearing screening test (otoacoustic emissions) bilaterally. Group mean data ($N = 20$ for each age group) are from the Sanford and Feeney (2008) study discussed earlier in this chapter.

Ambient ER data for S2 at one month of age and group data for one-month-olds are shown in Figure 7–13.

S2's ER data are about 20% higher than the mean for one-month-olds at frequencies from 0.3 to 2.0 kHz, with almost identical ER between 2.0 and 5.0 kHz. However, ER at 0.25 kHz is 35% higher for S2, than for group data.

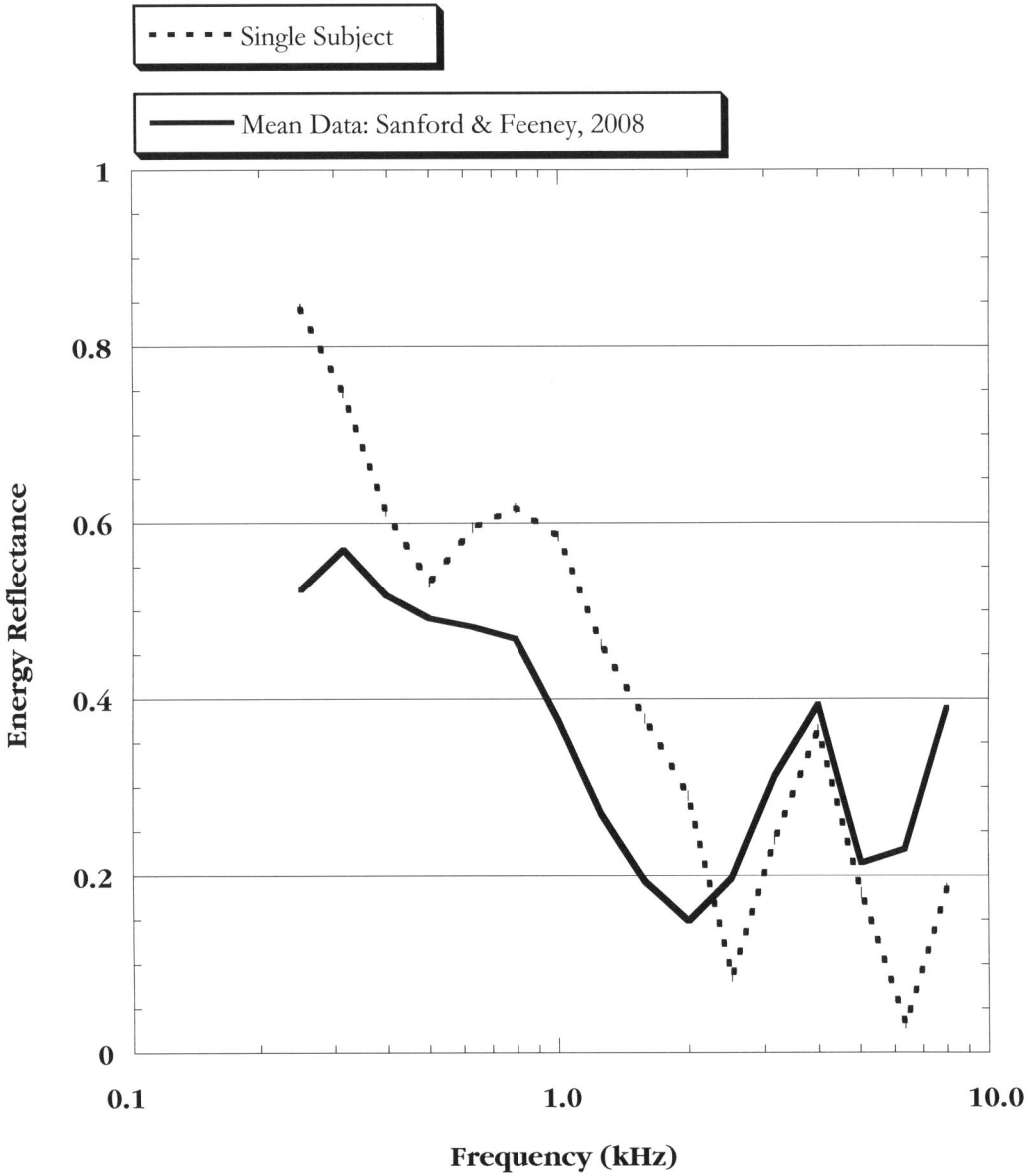

FIGURE 7–13. Single subject (S2—*dashed line*) and group mean (*solid line*) one-third-octave energy reflectance (ER) obtained at 1 month of age. Group mean data (*N* = 20 ears) from Sanford and Feeney (2008).

A similar pattern comparison of S2 and mean data can be made at 3 months as shown in Figure 7–14.

For both S2 and mean data, the "peaks" in ER at 4.0 kHz have diminished by 3 months of age. The greatest

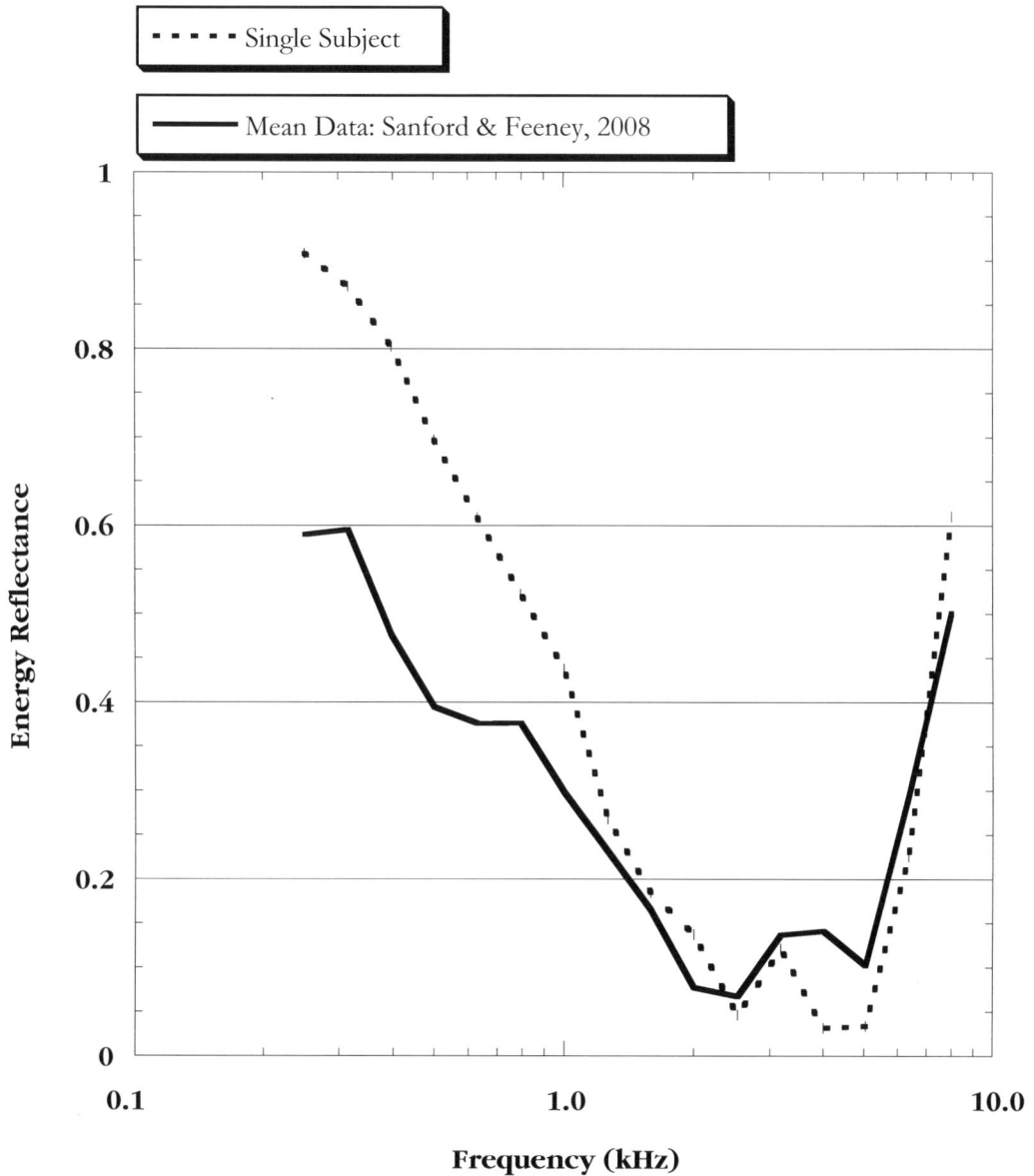

FIGURE 7–14. Single subject (S2—*dashed line*) and group mean (*solid line*) one-third-octave energy reflectance (ER) obtained at 3 months of age. Group mean data (*N* = 20 ears) from Sanford and Feeney (2008).

difference between S2 and the group mean is for frequencies below 1.0 kHz. Also ER at 0.25 kHz has increased for both S2 and group data by approximately 10%, keeping the relative differences in ER at 0.25 kHz about the same.

Data in Figure 7–15 shows S2's ER at 5 months of age and mean ER data at six months of age. S2's data are very similar to mean ER data across the entire frequency range. Some small differences are noted between 2.0 and 4.0 kHz and dif-

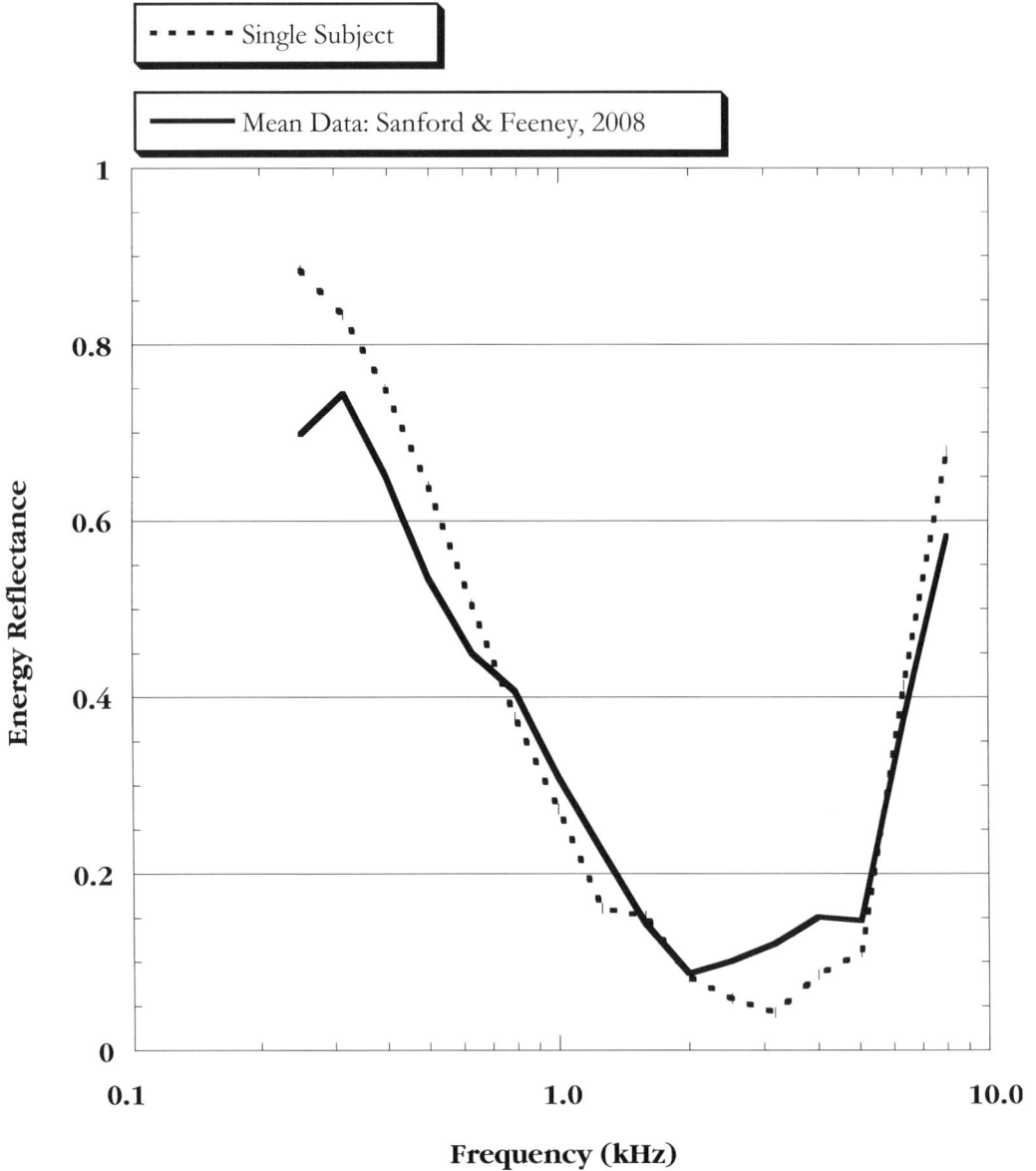

FIGURE 7–15. Single subject (S2—*dashed line*) and group mean (*solid line*) one-third-octave energy reflectance (ER) obtained at 5 and 6 months of age, respectively. Group mean data (*N* = 20 ears) from Sanford and Feeney (2008).

ferences observed at earlier ages for 0.25 kHz are still present, but less pronounced. As noted earlier, the lower reflectance for these lower frequencies for neonates and young infants may be the result of a more absorbent infant ear canals shunting low frequency energy, rather than a middle ear effect. (Keefe et al., 1993). The differences in ER for frequencies below 0.5 kHz for S2 and group data presented here may be highlighting individual variability in ear canal development. In the case of the S2, low frequency ER was adultlike at 3 months of age, whereas group data did not approach adultlike values until 6 months of age.

At 5.5 months of age, S2 presented with coldlike, upper respiratory problems and was diagnosed with otitis media with effusion (OME) in her left ear. She began a course of antibiotics shortly after diagnosis. Two days after OME diagnosis, ATF measurements were obtained for her left ear. Figure 7–16 shows ER data for S2's left ear at 5 months of age (pre-OME; dashed line) and at 5.5 months (present-OME diagnosis; square symbols).

ER measured in the OME condition at 5.5 months is only slightly higher at 0.25 kHz, but remains high (>0.65) out to 3.0 kHz. A sharp notch in ER is observed at 4.0 kHz. Then ER increases in a fashion similar to the pre-OME data

out to 8.0 kHz. Shown for comparison is the solid line in Figure 7–16 which represents mean ER acquired from four adult ears with OME (Feeney et al., 2003a). These adult data reveal a pattern of high ER with a high-frequency notch. Overall, this suggests that wideband ER is sensitive to middle ear effusion, which causes high ER results in the low- to mid-frequencies.

Case Study Summary

Examination of S2's data and group data suggests that significant changes in ER occur between 1 and 6 months of age, with less noticeable changes occurring between 3 and 6 months of age. Individual longitudinal data from S2 generally follow the trends observed in the group data. Examination of ATF data at more discrete ages and for ears with middle ear pathologies could help shed additional light on the time course of middle ear/ear canal developmental effects and potential usefulness of ATF data for diagnosing middle ear dysfunction in neonatal and infant populations.

Acknowledgments. The authors thank Lisa Hunter, Douglas Keefe, and Lynne Werner for sharing data from their studies.

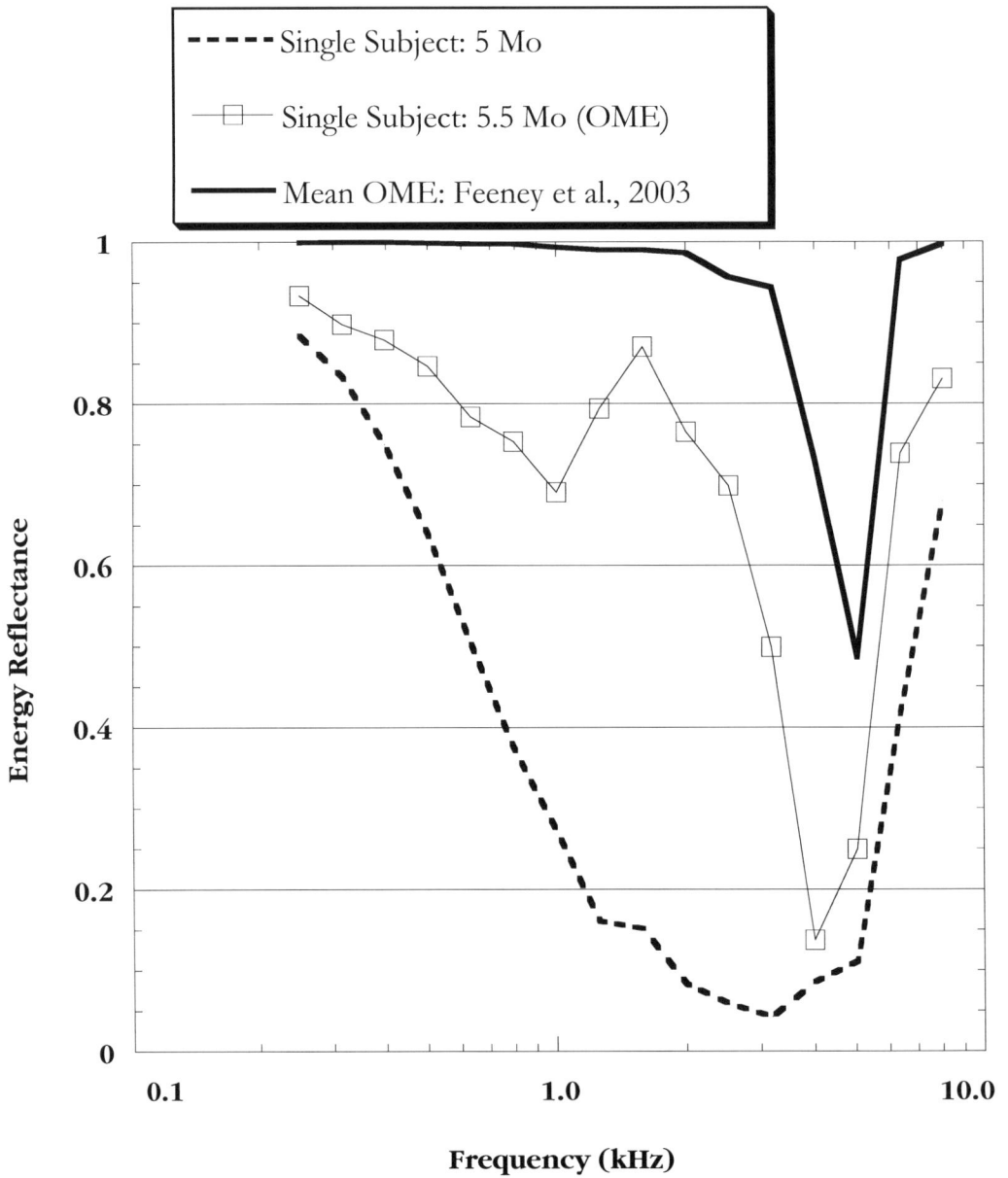

FIGURE 7–16. Single subject (S2) one-third-octave energy reflectance (ER) obtained at 5 months of age (*dashed line*) and at 5.5 months of age with a diagnosis of otitis media with effusion (*square symbols*). The solid black line represents mean ER data from 4 adult ears with otitis media with effusion from Feeney et al. (2003a).

REFERENCES

Abahazi, D. A., & Greenberg, H. J. (1977). Clinical acoustic reflex threshold measurements in infants. *Journal of Speech and Hearing Disorders, 42,* 515–519.

Allen, J. B. (1986). Measurement of eardrum acoustic impedance. In J. B. Allen, J. L. Hall, A. Hubbard, T. Neely, & A. Tubis (Eds.), *Peripheral auditory mechanisms* (pp. 44–51). New York, NY: Springer-Verlag.

Allen, J. B., Jeng, P. S., & Levitt, H. (2005). Evaluation of human middle ear function via an acoustic power assessment. *Journal of Rehabilitation Research and Development, 42,* 63–78.

American National Standards Institute (ANSI). (1987). *ANSI specifications for instruments to measure aural acoustic impedance and admittance (aural acoustic immittance).* ANSI S3.39–1987. New York, NY: Author.

Bennett, M. J. (1975). Acoustic impedance measurements with the neonate. *British Journal of Audiology, 9,* 117–124.

Boone, R.T., Bower, C. M., & Martin, P.F. (2005). Failed newborn hearing screens as presentation for otitis media with effusion in the newborn population. *International Journal of Pediatric Otorhinolaryngology, 69,* 393–397.

Chang, K. W., Vohr, B. R., Norton, S. J., & Lekas, M. D. (1993). External and middle ear status related to evoked otoacoustic emission in neonates. *Archives of Otolaryngology-Head and Neck Surgery, 119,* 276–282.

Doyle, K. J., Burggraaff, B., Fujikawa, S., & Kim, J. (1997). Neonatal hearing screening with otoscopy, auditory brain stem response, and otoacoustic emissions. *Otolaryngology-Head and Neck Surgery, 116,* 597–603.

Doyle, K. J., Kong, Y. Y., Strobel, K., Dallaire, P., & Ray, R. M. (2004). Neonatal middle ear effusion predicts chronic otitis media with effusion. *Otology and Neurotology, 25,* 318–322.

Feeney, M. P., Grant, I. L., & Marryott, L. P. (2003a). Wideband energy reflectance measurements in adults with middle ear disorders. *Journal of Speech, Language, and Hearing Research, 46,* 901–911.

Feeney, M. P., Grant, I. L., & Mills, D. M. (2009). Wideband energy reflectance measurements of ossicular chain discontinuity and repair in human temporal bone. *Ear and Hearing, 30,* 391–400.

Feeney M. P., & Keefe, D. H. (1999). Acoustic reflex detection using wide-band acoustic reflectance, admittance and power measurements. *Journal of Speech, Language and Hearing Research, 42,* 1029–1041.

Feeney, M. P., & Keefe, D. H. (2001). Estimating the acoustic reflex threshold from wideband measures of reflectance, admittance and power. *Ear and Hearing, 22,* 316–332.

Feeney, M. P., Keefe, D. H., & Marryott, L. P. (2003b). Contralateral acoustic reflex thresholds for tonal activators using wideband reflectance and admittance measurements. *Journal of Speech, Language and Hearing Research, 46,* 128–136.

Feeney, M. P., & Sanford, C. A. (2004). Age effects in the human middle ear: Wideband acoustical measures. *Journal of the Acoustical Society of America, 116,* 3546–3558.

Feeney, M. P., & Sanford, C. A. (2005). Detection of the acoustic stapedius reflex in infants using wideband energy reflectance and admittance. *Journal of the American Academy of Audiology, 16,* 278–290.

Holte, L., Cavanaugh, R. M., & Margolis, R. H. (1990). Ear-canal wall mobility and tympanometric shape in young infants. *Journal of Pediatrics, 117,* 77– 80.

Holte, L., Margolis, R. H., & Cavanaugh, R. M. (1991). Developmental changes in multi-frequency tympanograms. *Audiology, 30,* 1–24.

Hunter, L. L., Feeney, M. P., Lapsley Miller, J. A., Jeng, P. S., & Bohning, S. (2010). Wideband reflectance in newborns: Normative regions and relationship to hearing-screening results. *Ear and Hearing, 31,* 599–610.

Hunter, L. L., Tubaugh, L., Jackson, A., & Propes, S. (2008). Wideband middle ear power measurement in infants and children. *Journal of the American Academy of Audiology, 19,* 309–324.

Jerger, S., Jerger, J., Mauldin, L., & Segal, P. (1974). Studies in impedance audiometry II. Children less than 6 years old. *Archives of Otolaryngology, 99,* 1–9.

Joint Committee on Infant Hearing (JCIH). (2007). Year 2007 position statement: Principles and guidelines for early hearing detection and intervention programs. *Pediatrics, 120,* 898–921.

Keefe, D. H., Bulen, J. C., Arehart, K. H., & Burns, E. M. (1993). Ear-canal impedance and reflection coefficient in human infants and adults. *Journal of the Acoustical Society of America, 94,* 2617–2638.

Keefe, D. H., & Feeney, M. P. (2009). Principles of acoustic immittance and acoustic transfer functions. In J. Katz, L. Medwetsky, R. Burkhard, & L. J. Hood (Eds.), *Handbook of clinical audiology* (6th ed.). Baltimore, MD: Lippincott Williams & Wilkins.

Keefe, D. H., Fitzpatrick, D. F., Liu, Y., Sanford, C. A., & Gorga, M. P. (2010). Wideband acoustic reflex test in a test battery to predict middle-ear dysfunction. *Hearing Research, 263,* 52–65.

Keefe, D. H., Folsom, R. C., Gorga, M. P., Vohr, B. R., Bulen, J. C., & Norton, S. J. (2000). Identification of neonatal hearing impairment: Ear-canal measurements of acoustic admittance and reflectance in neonates. *Ear and Hearing, 21,* 443–461.

Keefe, D. H., Gorga, M. P., Neely, S. T., Zhao, F., & Vohr, B. (2003b). Ear-canal acoustic admittance and reflectance effects in human neonates. II. Predictions of middle ear dysfunction and sensorineural hearing loss. *Journal of the Acoustical Society of America, 113,* 407–422.

Keefe, D. H., Ling, R., & Bulen, J. C. (1992). Method to measure acoustic impedance and reflection coefficient. *Journal of the Acoustical Society of America, 91,* 470–485.

Keefe, D. H., & Simmons, J. L. (2003). Energy transmittance predicts conductive hearing loss in older children and adults. *Journal of the Acoustical Society of America, 114,* 3217–3238.

Keefe, D. H., Zhao, F., Neely, S. T., Gorga, M. P., & Vohr, B. R. (2003a). Ear-canal acoustic admittance and reflectance effects in human neonates. I. Predictions of otoacoustic emission and auditory brainstem responses. *Journal of the Acoustical Society of America, 113,* 389–406.

Keith, R. W. (1973). Impedance audiometry with neonates. *Archives of Otolaryngology, 97,* 465–467.

Kok, M. R., van Zanten, G. A., & Brocaar, M. P. (1992). Growth of evoked otoacoustic emissions during the first days postpartum: A preliminary report. *Audiology, 31,* 140–149.

Liu, Y-L., Sanford, C. A., Ellison, J. C., Fitzpatrick, D. F., Gorga, M. P., & Keefe, D. H. (2008). Wideband absorbance tympanometry using pressure sweeps: System development and results on adults with normal hearing. *Journal of the Acoustical Society of America, 124,* 3708–3719.

Margolis, R. H., Saly, G. L., & Keefe, D. H. (1999). Wideband reflectance tympanometry in normal adults. *Journal of* the *Acoustical Society of America, 106,* 265–280.

Meyer, S. E., Jardine, C. A., Deverson, W. (1997). Developmental changes in tympanometry: A case study. *British Journal of Audiology, 31,* 189–195.

Piskorski, P., Keefe, D. H., Simmons, J. L., & Gorga, M. P. (1999). Prediction of conductive hearing loss based on acoustic ear-canal response using a multivariate clinical decision theory. *Journal of the Acoustical Society of America, 105,* 1749–1764.

Rosenfeld, R. M., Culpepper, L., Doyle, K. J., Grundfast, K.M., Kenna, M.A., Hoberman, A., . . . Yawn, B. (2004). Clinical practice guideline: Otitis media with effusion. *Otolaryngology-Head and Neck Surgery, 130,* 95–118.

Ruah, C. B., Schachern, P. A., Zelterman, D., Paparella, M. M., & Yoon, T. H. (1991). Age-related morphologic changes in the human tympanic membrane. A light and electron microscopic study. *Archives of Otolaryngology Head and Neck Surgery, 117,* 627– 634.

Sanford, C. A., & Feeney, M. P. (2008). Effects of maturation on tympanometric wideband acoustic transfer functions in human infants. *Journal of the Acoustical Society of America, 124,* 2106–2122.

Sanford, C. A., Keefe, D. H., Liu, Y.-W., Fitzpatrick, D. F., McCreery, R., Lewis, D. E., & Gorga, M. P. (2009). Sound-conduction effects on DPOAE screening outcomes in newborn infants: Test performance of wideband acoustic transfer functions and 1.0-kHz tympanometry. *Ear and Hearing, 30,* 635–652.

Saunders, J. C., Kaltenback, J. A., & Relkin, E. M. (1983). The structural and functional development of the outer and middle ear. In R. Romand & M. R. Romand (Eds.), *Development of auditory and vestibular systems* (pp. 3–25). New York, NY: Academic Press.

Schairer, K. S., Ellison, J. C., Fitzpatrick, D., & Keefe, D. H. (2007). Wideband ipsilateral measurements of middle-ear muscle reflex thresholds in children and adults. *Journal of the Acoustical Society of America, 121,* 3607–3616.

Shahnaz, N. (2008). Wideband reflectance in neonatal intensive care units. *Journal of the American Academy of Audiology, 19,* 419–429.

Shahnaz, N., Bork, K., & Polka, L., Longridge, N., Bell, D., & Westerberg, B. D. (2009). Energy reflectance and tympanometry in normal and otosclerotic ears. *Ear and Hearing, 30,* 219–233.

Shahnaz, N., & Polka, L. (1997). Standard and multifrequency tympanometry in normal and otosclerotic ears. *Ear and Hearing, 18,* 326–341.

Shahnaz, N., & Polka, L. (2002). Distinguishing healthy from otosclerotic ears: Effect of probe-tone frequency on static immittance. *Journal of the American Academy of Audiology, 13,* 345–355.

Takahara, T., Sando, I., Hashida, Y., & Shibahara, Y. (1986). Mesenchyme remaining in human temporal bones. *Otolaryngology-Head and Neck Surgery, 95,* 349–357.

Vander Werff, K. R., Prieve, B. A., & Georgantas, L. M. (2007). Test-retest reliability of wideband reflectance measures in infants under screening and diagnostic test conditions. *Ear and Hearing, 28,* 669–681.

Weatherby, L. A., & Bennett, M. J. (1980). The neonatal acoustic reflex. *Scandinavian Audiology, 9,* 103–110.

Werner, L. A., Levi, E. C., & Keefe, D. H. (2010). Ear-canal wideband acoustic transfer functions of adults and two- to nine-month-old infants. *Ear and Hearing, 31,* 587–598.

CHAPTER 8

The Challenge of Assessing Middle Ear Function in Young Infants: Summary and Future Directions

JOSEPH KEI AND FEI ZHAO

INTRODUCTION

Assessment of middle ear function in young infants (aged 0 to 6 months) has been a real challenge. Since the 1970s, the use of conventional 226-Hz tympanometry has been found to be inaccurate in identifying middle ear problems in young infants. Since the 1980s, clinicians have prohibited its use with young infants. Clinicians then rely on auditory brainstem response (ABR) and otoacoustic emissions (OAEs) to identify conductive hearing loss in this young population. Although these physiologic measures provide useful clinical information, they are not direct measures of middle ear function.

Although preliminary studies provided evidence that alternative measures such as high frequency (>800 Hz) tympanometry, acoustic stapedial reflex test, multifrequency tympanometry, and wideband acoustic transfer functions may be useful, there have been little progress in developing these measures further until after 2000. To date, substantial research in this area has advanced knowledge about the usefulness or otherwise of these tests. This chapter provides a summary of various measures to assess the middle ear function in young infants. The advantages and disadvantages of these measures in assessing young infants are outlined. Future challenges and suggestions for clinical applications are delineated.

HIGH-FREQUENCY (1000 HZ) TYMPANOMETRY (HFT)

Since the introduction of HFT for assessing the middle ear function of young infants in 2003, the use of HFT in pediatric audiology clinics has gained popularity around the world. HFT has been found to be a useful technique for assessing the middle ear function of young infants aged between 0 and 6 months (Alaerts, Luts, & Wouters, 2007; Baldwin, 2006; Calandruccio, Fitzgerald, & Prieve, 2006; Kei et al., 2003; Margolis, Bass-Ringdahl, Hanks, Holte, & Zapala, 2003; Mazlan, Kei, Hickson, Gavranich, & Linning, 2009c). Although multifrequency techniques (discussed in Chapters 5, 6, and 7) may provide a comprehensive view of the middle ear dynamics of young infants, HFT offers a quick and direct measure of middle ear function for this young population. The advantages of the HFT include:

■ *Good test performance*—Using otoacoustic emission (OAE) test outcomes as a gold standard, the sensitivity and specificity of HFT have been reported to be 0.57 to 0.91 and 0.5 to 0.95, respectively (Margolis et al., 2003; Swanepoel, Werner, Hugo, Louw, Owen, & Swanepoel, 2007). Baldwin (2006) obtained very high HFT test performance with a sensitivity

of 0.99 and specificity of 0.89, using ABR outcomes as a gold standard.

■ *High test-retest reliability*—The HFT test has been found to be a reliable test for newborns and 6-week-old infants, with no significant difference in findings across test and retest conditions. The correlation coefficients across the test-retest conditions for the peak compensated static admittance with baseline compensation and with component compensation at 200 daPa for newborns were 0.89 and 0.86, respectively (Mazlan, Kei, Hickson, Gavranich, & Linning, 2010). The corresponding correlation coefficients for the 6-week-old infants were greater than those for the newborns (Mazlan et al., 2010).

■ *Time efficient*—HFT is a quick test that can be completed within 5 minutes for a quiet infant.

■ *Uncomplicated test findings*—Kei et al. (2003) found that 92% of healthy newborn infants showed a single positive-peaked admittance tympanogram. Hence, the interpretation of HFT findings is much simplified in comparison to the use of the Vanhuyse, Creten, and Van Camp (1975) model in interpreting the conductance and susceptance tympanograms. As regards the interpretation of HFT findings, Baldwin (2006) adopted an approach based on the morphology of HFT tracings: a single positive peak indicates a "pass," and a flat or negative peak indicates a "refer." Margolis et al. (2003) and Kei, Mazlan, Hickson, Gavranich, and Linning (2007) used an approach based on both morphology and a quantitative measure of the peak compensated static admittance.

▧ *Availability of normative data*—Normative data are available for infants aged from 0 to 4 weeks (e.g., Calandruccio et al., 2006; Kei et al., 2003; Margolis et al., 2003; Mazlan et al., 2009c).

Despite the advantages of HFT listed above, there are still unresolved issues regarding HFT measurements. First, there is no universally agreed method for interpreting HFT results. Currently, the morphology approach and morphology plus quantitative measures approach are being used in clinics. It is not certain which approach has a higher sensitivity and specificity in diagnosing middle ear dysfunction. As regards the quantitative measures, which test parameter or a combination of parameters is more sensitive to middle ear dysfunction in young infants? If the peak compensated static admittance (admittance of the middle ear) were an important test parameter, should compensation be made for the susceptance component only, or both the susceptance and conductance components? Should the compensation be made at 200 daPa or at −400 daPa? What is the rationale for compensating at 200 daPa or −400 daPa?

Second, there is no calibration standard which utilizes a probe tone of 1 kHz for the HFT equipment. Presently, it is based on measurements of acoustic admittance magnitude and phase angle using a 226-Hz tone in a 2-mL calibration cavity. There is an assumption that if the calibration works well for the 226-Hz tone, it will also work for the 1-kHz-probe tone. However, this assumption has not been validated. If the calibration is not valid, all measurements will be inaccurate. Perhaps, calibration could be one of the confounding factors leading to differences in normative data recorded by different HFT devices. More research is needed to validate this proposition.

Third, the instrumentation and test procedure for the HFT have not been standardized. For example, the GSI TymStar delivers a probe tone of 1 kHz at 85 dB SPL, whereas the Madsen Otoflex 100 delivers the tone at 75 dB SPL. Would 85 dB SPL be better than the 75 dB SPL when it applies to the tiny ears of young infants?

Last, the test performance of HFT has not been accurately measured. Previous studies evaluating the test performance of HFT were based on the outcomes of the OAE test. However, the literature shows that some children with subtle middle ear dysfunctions can pass the OAE test (e.g., Driscoll, Kei, & McPherson, 2001). In future studies, a different gold standard based on the test outcomes of a combination of tests, which are sensitive to subtle middle ear dysfunctions, may be used.

In summary, HFT has an important role to play in assessing the middle ear function of young infants. There is clear evidence that the test performance of HFT in identifying middle ear disorders is higher than that of 226-Hz or 678-Hz tympanometry. However, there are still issues with the measurement and interpretation of HFT results. These issues need to be addressed by researchers and clinicians in collaboration with the industry (manufacturers of audiologic equipment).

ACOUSTIC STAPEDIAL REFLEX TEST

The acoustic stapedial reflex (ASR) test has many useful applications including the detection of middle ear problems, cochlear and retrocochlear lesions (Margolis, 1993). Although a complete test protocol involves the elicitation of the ASR by both contralateral and ipsilateral stimulation methods, the detection of middle ear dysfunction in young infants can best be achieved through ipsilateral stimulation alone. The ASR test is particularly sensitive to middle ear pathology because the elicitation of the ASR is affected by both the stimulus ear effects and the probe ear effects of conductive disorders (Gelfand, 2009).

The ipsilateral ASR test can be used as an adjunct clinical tool to the existing screening instrument such as automated ABR or OAEs in universal newborn hearing screening (UNHS) programs. Given that the majority of infants who are referred by UNHS programs have conductive hearing loss, the use of the ASR to distinguish conductive from sensorineural hearing impairment will streamline the referral procedure for better management of infants. Those infants with suspected permanent sensorineural hearing loss will require investigation using the ABR test, whereas those with suspected conductive pathology will require follow-up appointments using specialized tests for evaluating middle ear function. This streamlining of referrals will reduce the demand and waiting list for the ABR test and will result in a huge reduction in service cost to the national health care system.

In summary, the advantages of the ASR test are:

- *High test performance*—Using OAE test outcomes as a gold standard, the test performance of the ASR/HFT combination in identifying middle ear fluid in young infants was found to be higher than that of the HFT alone (Swanepoel et al., 2007).

- *High test-retest reliability*—The ASR test has been found to be a reliable test for newborns with no significant difference in ASR thresholds across test and retest conditions for the 0.5, 2, and 4 kHz, and broadband noise stimuli. High correlation coefficients for the ASR thresholds across test-retest conditions were obtained (Kei, in press; Mazlan, Kei, & Hickson, 2009a). The reliability of the ASR test for 6-week-old infants was as good as for newborns (Mazlan et al., 2009b).

- *Time efficient*—The ASR is a quick test which follows the HFT test. The test can be completed in 5 min for a quiet infant.

- *Interpretation of test findings*—Unlike the HFT test, ASR test findings are simple to interpret. The possible outcomes of the ASR test are absent ASR, raised ASR threshold or normal ASR threshold. The normal range for each stimulus can be established based on normative data.

Although the ASR test is valuable as an alternative instrument to detect middle ear problems, there are limitations in its application to young infants. First, the involuntary movement of the infant during testing may create artifacts in the tracing which may be interpreted as an ASR response. Great care should be taken to distinguish movement artifacts from genuine ASR responses. Second, clinicians should be aware that an ASR response obtained from a young infant may be considered when the change in admittance, in either the upward (increase) or downward (decrease) direction, exceeds a certain cutoff value. It is necessary to check if the change in admittance increases with increasing stimulus intensity to distinguish a genuine ASR response from an artifact. Third, there presently is no unanimous agreement on the minimum change in admittance to be considered an ASR response. It varies from 0.02 to 0.04 mmho (Kei, in press; Kei et al., 2007; Mazlan et al., 2009a; Swanepoel et al., 2007). Last, there is some evidence that ASR threshold may be a function of age within the first few weeks of life. For instance, Mazlan et al. (2007) found that the mean ASR threshold increased from 73.1 dB HL for newborns to 79.6 dB HL for infants aged 6 to 7 weeks. Given this change in ASR threshold with age, there is a need to establish age-specific normative ASR data for infants in their first 6 months of life. However, normative ASR data for other age brackets have not been developed. More research in this area is warranted.

SWEEP FREQUENCY IMPEDANCE (SFI) TEST

The SFI meter, developed by Hiroshi Wada and his colleagues in the early 1990s, provides useful information about the characteristics of middle ear dynamics, including the resonance frequency of the middle ear and its mobility in terms of changes in sound pressure (ΔSPL) in the resonance frequency region. Unlike the multifrequency tympanometric technique, the SFI provides a distinctive way to measure the resonance frequency and mobility of the middle ear. Besides, the SFI measurements can be validated by theoretical data.

The middle ear dynamic characteristics of some disorders, as revealed by SFI findings, are described below:

- In patients with retracted tympanic membrane (TM) and tympanosclerosis, their SFI results indicate high resonance frequency and significantly reduced ΔSPL at normal static pressure, consistent with a high-stiffness middle ear.

- In patients with TM perforation, sound-pressure variation (ΔSPL) is larger than that of a normal-hearing subject. In addition, a frequency notch may be observed below 1.0 kHz.

- In patients with severe secretory otitis media, SFI findings indicate high resonance frequency with significantly reduced ΔSPL at normal static pressure, consistent with high stiffness in the middle ear.

■ The dynamic characteristics in patients with otosclerosis involving the stapes footplate vary depending on the pathologic stage of the disease. Their SFI results are generally in agreement with high stiffness in the middle ear, having a high resonance frequency and significantly reduced ΔSPL.

■ Patients with ossicular chain separation have a low resonance frequency and increased ΔSPL at normal static pressure, consistent with low stiffness middle ear status.

In summary, the SFI has been found to provide useful clinical information for identifying middle ear disorders such as ossicular chain fixation, ossicular chain separation, ototis media with effusion, and tympanic membrane aberrations and perforation. The SFI test is more sensitive to ossicular chain disorders than conventional 226-Hz tympanometry (Wada, Koike, & Kobayashi, 1998; Zhao, Wada, Koike, Ohyama, Kawase, & Stephens, 2002, 2003).

Despite these advantages, there are limitations in SFI measurements and its interpretation. Although the ΔSPL reflects middle ear mobility, it is not independent of the resonance frequency. That is, when the resonance frequency increases (e.g., close to 2.0 kHz), the ΔSPL decreases and vice versa. In view of this characteristic feature, the diagnosis of middle ear disorders may be affected. For instance, a normally hearing adult with a higher than normal resonance frequency (e.g., 1.6 kHz) and reduced ΔSPL may be interpreted as having a high-stiffness middle ear condition. In addition, there is a certain degree of overlap in terms of middle ear dynamic

characteristics between individuals with normal middle ear function and those with middle ear disorders. For an accurate diagnosis, the SFI results must be interpreted in conjunction with the results of other tests including case history, otoscopy, and audiometric measures.

As discussed in Chapter 6, the SFI results obtained from healthy neonates are clearly different from those of adults in that there are two variations (inflections) located at about 0.3 and 1.2 kHz in the SFI curve at normal static pressure (around 0 daPa). This indicates the possibility of having two vibrating elements in the neonatal external and middle ear. It is postulated that the vibrating element located at 1.2 kHz may be related to the resonance of the middle ear (Wada & Kobayashi, 1990), while the other vibrating element which occurs around 0.3 kHz may be related to the external ear canal being more flaccid than that of the adult.

There are two important issues regarding the interpretation of SFI findings obtained from neonates. First, the origin of the vibrating element that occurs around 0.3 kHz is still unclear. What is the significance of having this vibrating element? Will the frequency and ΔSPL change with age? At what age will this vibrating element disappear? What is the theoretical explanation behind this vibrating element? Second, the variation of the SFI curve located at 1.2 kHz covers a wide frequency range and the inflection is not as distinct as that for adults. This may involve a large error in measuring the resonance frequency and ΔSPL.

At present, the SFI device has not been commercialized, even though many efforts have been made for its further development and clinical applications in recent years. Further research needs to be done to investigate middle ear function in healthy neonates and young infants with middle ear disorders.

WIDEBAND ACOUSTIC TRANSFER FUNCTIONS (ATF)

A wideband ATF measures the incident and the reflected sound energy from the tympanic membrane using a wideband click or chirp. From these measurements, it is possible to measure the ATF absorbance which represents the proportion of sound energy absorbed by the middle ear. Absorbance varies from 1.0 (total absorption) to 0.0 (no absorption) depending on how much energy is absorbed by the middle ear. Energy reflectance (ER), defined as "1–Absorbance," is frequently used in research.

The ATF measuring system has been used to evaluate middle ear disorders in adults, children, and young infants. There are special features in ATF that are not shared by single-frequency tympanometry techniques (Feeney, Grant, & Marryott, 2003; Keefe, Ling, & Bulen, 1992; Margolis, Saly, & Keefe, 1999; Zhao, Lowe, Meredith, & Rhodes, 2008; Zhao, Meredith, Wotherspoon, & Rhodes, 2007). First, ATF provides measurements of the transfer function over a wide frequency range (0.25 to 8 kHz); Second, ATF measurements are more closely related to hearing sensitivity than measures of immittances. Last, ATF is less sensitive than immittance measures to probe position and standing waves in the ear canal. Because the measurement of ATF is simple, fast, objective, reproducible, and noninvasive, and because ATF results are associated with certain types of middle ear pathologies, ATF has great potential for identifying middle ear disorders.

Various studies have investigated the clinical importance of ATF in the detection of middle ear pathologies that are not readily detected by single-frequency (226 Hz or 1 kHz) tympanometry. Table 8–1 summarizes seven studies using ATF to evaluate middle ear function in different age groups. As shown in this table, earlier studies showed ER changes in a small number of cases with various middle ear pathological changes (Feeney et al. 2003; Hunter & Margolis, 1997; Margolis et al., 1999), whereas other studies focused on investigating specific middle ear pathological conditions with relatively large sample sizes (Beers, Shahnaz, Westerberg, & Kozak, 2010; Hunter, Bagger-Sjöbäck, & Lundberg, 2008; Shahnaz, Bork, Polka, Longridge, Bell, & Westerberg, 2009a; Shahnaz, Longridge, & Bell, (2009b). Some studies provided evidence that ATF was more sensitive than 226-Hz or 1-kHz tympanometry in identifying middle ear pathologies, such as otitis media with effusion and otosclerosis, (e.g., Hunter et al., 2008; Shahnaz et al., 2009a). These results are in keeping with the results of Sanford, Keefe, Liu, Fitzpatrick, McCreery, Lewis, and Gorga (2009) discussed in Chapter 7. In general, all these studies demonstrated distinctive ATF results, depending on the nature and extent of the pathological conditions.

TABLE 8–1. Summary of ATF Findings from Seven Studies Published During the Period from 1997 to 2010

Study	Subjects and Sample	Summary of the Main Results	Evaluation
Hunter & Margolis (1997)	7 case studies including; otitis media, eustachian tube dysfunction, typmanosclerosis, cholesteatoma, perforation.	An otitis media case revealed normal static admittance with negative middle ear pressure using 226-Hz tympanometry. There were abnormally high ER values at frequencies between 1.2 and 4 kHz, followed by a deep notch between 4 and 6 kHz.	**Strengths:** Provided overview information on various middle ear disorders, together with other audiometric information. **Weaknesses:** An early study using ATF with a limited sample size and comparison with adult normative data.
Margolis et al. (1999)	10-year-old male with otitis media	Tympanometry revealed left negative middle ear pressure. Reflectance results showed abnormally high ER values up to 4000 Hz, when pressurized to compensate for the negative middle ear pressure.	**Strengths:** Provided overview information on multiple frequency tympanometry, together with knowledge on Vanhuyse mathematic model. **Weaknesses:** An early study using ATF with a limited sample size and comparison with adult normative data.

Study	Subjects and Sample	Summary of the Main Results	Evaluation
Feeney et al. (2003)	40 control adult subjects (age range = 19 to 24 yr) and 10 adult cases (age range = 21 to 65 yr) including: SNHL (2 ears) OME (4 ears) OTO (2 ears) DIS (1 ear) HYP (2 ears) PERF (2 ears) NEG (2 ears)	Normal reflectance patterns were found with the SNHL ears. OME ears had abnormally high ER values up to 4 kHz with a deep notch centered at 5 kHz; OTO ears fell within the 95th percentile of normative data except for abnormally high ER values between 250–1189 Hz and 5993–7551 Hz; DIS & HYP ears fell within the 95th percentile of normative data except for abnormally low ER values approximately between 300–1000 Hz and abnormally high ER values approximately between 3000–5000 Hz; PERF ears mainly showed abnormally low ER values up to 841 Hz; NEG ears were similar to SNHL ears except for abnormally high ER values at approximately 250–1000 Hz.	**Strengths:** First comprehensive study providing information on ER changes in various middle ear disorders. **Weaknesses:** Normative data was obtained from a significantly younger group. Limited sample size in each individual middle ear disorder group.
Hunter et al. (2008)	17 cleft palate children with OME aged 9 weeks to 25 months, 97 control subjects aged between 3 days and 47 months were used from a separate study.	Average ER for the cleft palate children with OME was abnormally high (i.e., mean ± 1 SD) at the frequencies between 1 and 4 kHz. The largest difference was found at 2 kHz, where the averaged ER reached 1.0, compared to 0.23 obtained from healthy children. Sensitivity of OAE (88%) and ATF (82%) were greater than 226-Hz (67%) and 1000-Hz tympanometry (73%).	**Strengths:** Provided information related to sensitivity of the ATF by comparing with conventional and high-frequency tympanometry, together with DPOAE results. **Weaknesses:** Lack of surgical gold standard validation of OME. Limited statistical analysis.

continues

TABLE 8–1. *continued*

Study	Subjects and Sample	Summary of the Main Results	Evaluation
Feeney et al. (2009)	Five fresh human temporal bones.	Disarticulating the ossicular chain: a deep ER notch was found between 561 and 841 Hz. After repairing the disarticulated ossicular chain, the low frequency notch in ER disappeared. Theoretical analysis using a middle ear model showed that the low-frequency notch in ER mainly occurred at the resonance frequency in the condition of ossicular chain separation. A reduction in stapes displacement was found in the condition of the ossicular discontinuity using laser Doppler vibrometry.	**Strengths:** Other methods (simple series impedance model, laser Doppler vibrometry) were used to compare the changes obtained from ATF for the purpose of cross-evaluation. **Weaknesses:** Nonclinical population.
Shahnaz et al. (2009a)	28 patients diagnosed with otosclerosis. Age range = 24–56 yrs (mean = 41.6 yrs). 62 control subjects. Age range = 20–32 yrs (mean = 25.7 yrs).	71% of the otosclerotic ears showed that ER was higher than the 90th percentile of the normal ears below 1 kHz. Only a small proportion of the otosclerotic ears (10%) had higher ER values than the normal ears above 1500 Hz. The averaged ER in the otosclerotic ears was statistically higher than that in the normal ears between 400 and 1000 Hz. When using the 90th percentile for all frequencies as a normal criterion, 82% of otosclerotic ears were identified. ROC analysis revealed that ATF was useful in differentiating otosclerotic ears from normal ears by providing supplementary information to conventional tympanometry.	**Strengths:** Relatively large sample and control group. Examined sensitivity and specificity of ATF by comparison with 226 Hz tympanometry. **Weaknesses:** Normative data was obtained from significantly younger group.

Study	Subjects and Sample	Summary of the Main Results	Evaluation
Shahnaz et al. (2009b)	15 patients diagnosed with otosclerosis. Age range = 24–56 yrs (mean = 44 yrs). 62 control subjects. Age range = 20–32 yrs (mean = 25.7 yrs).	A deep notch between 700 and 1000 Hz in ER was found in the majority of the subjects, followed by a small increase in ER between 2 and 4 kHz after the surgery. Compared with hearing thresholds, there was a positive trend between ER changes in low frequencies and hearing improvement in both low- and high-frequency bands.	**Strengths:** ER changes were compared with the improvement in pure-tone hearing thresholds. **Weaknesses:** No conventional tympanometry results postoperatively.
Beers et al. (2010)	64 cases aged 3–12 yr (mean = 6.3 yrs), including: Subgroup 1: 21 (30 ears), mild negative pressure; Subgroup 2: 18 (24 ears), severe negative pressure; Subgroup 3: 25 (42 ears), OME. Control group consisted of 78 children aged 5–7 yrs (mean = 6.15 yrs).	Significant differences in ER levels across a wide range of frequencies between control group and three other diseased groups. ER levels measured from the group with mild negative middle ear pressure did not differ significantly from those obtained from the group with severe negative middle ear pressure at any frequency. ER at 1250 Hz had the largest ROC curve (sensitivity of 96% and specificity of 95%). Comparison of ROC curves between ATF at 1250 Hz and static admittance at 226-Hz probe-tone frequency revealed significantly better test performance for ATF in distinguishing between healthy ears and OME.	**Strengths:** Relatively large sample and control group. Examined sensitivity and specificity of ATF when compared with 226 Hz tympanometry outcomes. **Weaknesses:** Variability in age range between experimental and control groups.

ATF = acoustic transfer function; DIS = disarticulation; DPOAE = distortion product otoacoustic emissions; ER = energy reflectance; HYP = hypermobile tympanic membrane; NEG = negative middle ear pressure; OME = otitis media with effusion; OTO = otosclerosis; PERF = perforated tympanic membrane; ROC = receiver operating characteristics; SNHL = sensorineural hearing loss.

The strengths and apparent weaknesses of these studies are also delineated. For example, the results obtained from those early studies were based on limited samples, which are less powerful to provide sufficient evidence on the accuracy of ATF measurements. Although the studies with relatively large sample sizes provided useful information on the sensitivity and specificity of the ATF, there were limitations in experimental design. For instance, age- and gender-matched controls were not always available for comparison with experimental subjects. More importantly, the gold standard for validation of the pathologic conditions, especially in young infants, was not ideal. Also, establishing a gold standard based on surgery findings was not viable.

Although ATF has been shown to provide clinical information about the status of the middle ear, there are challenges in various aspects of ATF assessments. First, the ATF equipment is presently not available on the commercial market, although a research version of the device, developed by Interacoustics A/S, is being tested by researchers around the world. At present, many clinicians are not aware of the function of ATF and its application to identification of middle ear disorders. Second, large scale studies are required to provide detailed clinical data on patients with various middle ear pathologies. Third, large scale studies comparing ATF outcomes with a more appropriate gold standard to establish the sensitivity and specificity of ATF are needed. Normally hearing subjects with age and gender matched to the experimental

subjects are required. Last, ATF findings obtained from healthy neonates show lower reflectance in the low frequencies than that from adults. This difference in ATF findings is attributed to a more absorbent infant ear canal shunting low frequency energy, rather than a middle ear effect (Keefe et al., 1992). Can the neonatal ATF results be predicted using a theoretical approach? Successful application of a theoretical approach may advance knowledge in understanding the dynamical behavior of a neonate's external and middle ear.

CONCLUSIONS AND FUTURE RESEARCH

The primary aim of this book is to provide an up-to-date reference source in the field of middle ear assessment for young infants. By drawing on the knowledge and expertise of experts from various countries, this book has provided details of the entire collection of audiological tests of middle ear function for young infants, including HFT, ASR, multifrequency tympanometry, SFI, and ATF tests. These tests are in different stages of development and practice. Although the HFT and ASR tests are more frequently used with young infants in clinics, the SFI and ATF tests are still restricted to the laboratory as they are not yet commercially available.

Although the feasibility and applicability of the above tests have been established, there are unresolved issues with calibration, test procedures, and interpretation of findings in some of these tests. Once the calibration and test procedures are standardized, the interpretation of findings (including pass and fail criteria) will be consistent across clinics and across countries. Researchers and manufacturers of equipment need to address these issues as a priority.

The acoustic dynamical behavior of the middle ear in neonates, as revealed by SFI results, may be predicted using a theoretical approach. This approach, based on a mathematical model of the mechanics and physical properties of the middle ear, has been successful in predicting SFI results for adults (Wada & Kobayashi, 1990). Given that the test results obtained from healthy neonates are different from those obtained from adults, it may be possible in future to apply a similar theoretical approach to predict SFI results for healthy neonates. This mathematical model of the dynamics of the middle ear of neonates cannot be built without realizing the neonates' anatomical and physiological characteristics as discussed in Chapter 1. By the same token, it is possible in the near future to establish a theoretical model to predict ATF findings in neonates. Research in this area of modeling has already started (e.g., Feeney, Grant, & Mills, 2009). Further research in modeling is necessary to understand the theory behind the experimental results.

Each test of middle ear function for young infants has its merits and limitations. It would be advantageous to compare results obtained from different tests on the same patient with a specific disorder. Large-scale studies comparing outcomes from different tests using

an appropriate gold standard to establish the test performance of these tests are needed. The gold standard may be based on the outcomes of a combination of tests rather than the otoacoustic emission test outcomes alone, given that surgery outcomes are not a viable option.

In conclusion, middle ear assessment in young infants is essential. Many measures of auditory function such as OAEs and ABR are affected by inefficient transmission of sound through the middle ear. Without knowing the dynamic characteristics of the middle ear with or without a disorder, it is not possible to interpret OAE and ABR results with accuracy. This book has provided five different measures to evaluate the function of the middle ear. Clinicians must realize the potential of each measure to ascertain the status of the middle ear. To this end, large-scale studies targeting a particular disorder using normally hearing subjects and patients with that disorder are required, not only to establish the sensitivity and specificity of the measure for the disorder, but also provide detailed clinical data on patients at various stages of that disorder. It is important to disseminate the research findings widely so that clinicians have ready access to these data.

REFERENCES

Alaerts, J., Luts, H., & Wouters, J. (2007). Evaluation of middle ear function in young children: Clinical guidelines for the use of 226- and 1000-Hz tympanometry. *Otology and Neuro-Otology, 28,* 727–732.

Baldwin, M. (2006). Choice of probe tone and classification of trace patterns in tympanometry undertaken in early infancy. *International Journal of Audiology, 45,* 417–427.

Beers, A. N., Shahnaz, N., Westerberg, B. D., & Kozak, F. K. (2010).Wideband reflectance in normal Caucasian and Chinese school-aged children and in children with otitis media with effusion. *Ear and Hearing, 31,* 221–233.

Calandruccio, L., Fitzgerald, T. S., & Prieve, B. A. (2006). Normative multifrequency tympanometry in infants and toddlers. *Journal of the American Academy of Audiology 17,* 470–480.

Driscoll, C., Kei, J., & McPherson, B. (2001). Outcomes of transient evoked otoacoustic emission testing in six-year-old school children: A comparison with pure tone screening and tympanometry. *International Journal of Pediatric Otorhinolaryngology, 57,* 67–76.

Feeney, M. P., Grant, I. L., & Marryott, L. P. (2003). Wideband energy reflectance measurements in adults with middle-ear disorders. *Journal of Speech, Language, and Hearing Research, 46,* 901–911.

Feeney, M. P., Grant, I. L., & Mills, D. M. (2009). Wideband energy reflectance measurements of ossicular chain discontinuity and repair in human temporal bone. *Ear and Hearing, 30,* 391–400.

Gelfand, S.A. (2009). The acoustic reflex. In J. Katz, L. Medwetsky, R. Burkard, & L. Hood (Eds.), *Handbook of clinical audiology* (6th ed.). Baltimore, MD: Lippincott Williams & Wilkins.

Hunter, L. L., Bagger-Sjöbäck, D., & Lundberg, M. (2008). Wideband reflectance associated with otitis media in infants and children with cleft palate. *International Journal of Audiology, 47,* S57–S61.

Hunter, L. L., & Margolis, R. H. (1997). Effects of tympanic membrane abnor-

malities on auditory function. *Journal of the American Academy of Audiology, 8,* 431–446.

Keefe, D. H., Ling, R., & Bulen, J. C. (1992). Method to measure acoustic impedance and reflection coefficient. *Journal of the Acoustical Society of America, 91,* 470–485.

Kei, J. (in press). Acoustic stapedial reflexes in healthy neonates: Normative data and test-retest reliability. *Journal of the American Academy of Audiology.*

Kei, J., Allison-Levick, J., Dockray, J., Harrys, R., Kirkegard, C., Wong, J., . . . & Tudehope, D. (2003). High frequency (1000 Hz) tympanometry in normal neonates. *Journal of the American Academy of Audiology, 14,* 20–28.

Kei, J., Mazlan, R., Hickson, L., Gavranich, J., & Linning, R. (2007). Measuring middle ear admittance in newborns using 1000 Hz tympanometry: A comparison of methodologies. *Journal of the American Academy of Audiology, 18,* 739–748.

Margolis, R. H. (1993). Detection of hearing impairment with the acoustic stapedius reflex. *Ear and Hearing, 14,* 3–10.

Margolis, R. H., Bass-Ringdahl, S., Hanks, W. D., Holte, L., & Zapala, D. A. (2003). Tympanometry in newborn infants—1 kHz norms. *Journal of the American Academy of Audiology, 14,* 383–391.

Margolis, R. H., Saly, G. L., & Keefe, D. H. (1999). Wideband reflectance tympanometry in normal adults. *Journal of the Acoustical Society of America, 106,* 265–280.

Mazlan, R., Kei, J., & Hickson, L. (2009a). Test-retest reliability of acoustic reflex testing in healthy newborns. *Ear and Hearing, 30,* 295–301.

Mazlan, R., Kei, J., Hickson, L., Curtain, S., Baker, G., Jarman, K., Glyde, H., Gavranich, J., & Linning, R. (2009b). Test-retest reliability of acoustic reflex test in 6-week-old healthy infants. *Australian and New Zealand Journal of Audiology, 31,* 25–32.

Mazlan, R., Kei, J., Hickson, L., Gavranich, J., & Linning, R. (2009c). High frequency (1000 Hz) tympanometry findings in newborns: Normative data using a component compensated admittance approach. *Australian and New Zealand Journal of Audiology, 31,* 15–24.

Mazlan, R., Kei, J., Hickson, L., Gavranich, J., & Linning, R. (2010). Test-retest reproducibility of the 1000 Hz tympanometry in newborn and 6-week-old healthy infants. *International Journal of Audiology, 49,* 815–822.

Mazlan, R., Kei, J., Hickson, L., Stapleton, C., Grant, S., Lim, S., . . . Linning, R. (2007). High frequency immittance findings: Newborn versus 6-week-old infants. *International Journal of Audiology, 46,* 711–717.

Sanford, C. A., Keefe, D. H., Liu, Y.-W., Fitzpatrick, D. F ., McCreery, R., Lewis, D. E., & Gorga, M. P. (2009). Sound-conduction effects on DPOAE screening outcomes in newborn infants: Test performance of wideband acoustic transfer functions and 1.0-kHz tympanometry. *Ear and Hearing, 30,* 635–652.

Shahnaz, N., Bork, K., Polka, L., Longridge, N., Bell, D., & Westerberg, B. D. (2009a). Energy reflectance and tympanometry in normal and otosclerotic ears. *Ear and Hearing, 30,* 219–233.

Shahnaz, N., Longridge, N., & Bell, D. (2009b). Wideband energy reflectance patterns in preoperative and postoperative otosclerotic ears. *International Journal of Audiology, 48,* 240–247.

Swanepoel, D. W., Werner, S., Hugo, R., Louw, B., Owen, R., & Swanepoel, A. (2007). High frequency immittance for neonates: A normative study. *Acta Otolaryngologica, 127,* 49–56.

Vanhuyse, V. J., Creten, W. L., & Van Camp, K. J. (1975). On the W-notching of tympanogram. *Scandinavian Audiology, 4,* 45–50.

Wada, H., & Kobayashi, T. (1990). Dynamical behavior of middle ear: Theoretical study corresponding to measurement results obtained by a newly developed measuring apparatus. *Journal of the American Academy of Audiology, 87,* 237–245.

Wada, H., Koike, T., & Kobayashi, T. (1998). Clinical applicability of the sweep frequency measuring apparatus for diagnosis of middle ear diseases. *Ear and Hearing, 19,* 240–249.

Zhao, F., Lowe, G., Meredith, R., & Rhodes, A. (2008). The characteristics of otoreflectance and its test-retest reliability. *Asia Pacific Journal of Speech, Language, and Hearing, 11,* 1–7.

Zhao, F., Meredith, R., Wotherspoon, N., & Rhodes, A. (2007). Towards an understanding of middle ear mechanism using otoreflectance: The characteristics of energy reflectance. *Proceedings of the 4th Symposium on Middle Ear Mechanics and Otology,* pp. 60–68.

Zhao, F., Wada, H., Koike, T., Ohyama, K., Kawase, T., & Stephens, D. (2002). Middle ear dynamic characteristics in patients with otosclerosis. *Ear and Hearing, 23,* 150–158.

Zhao, F., Wada, H., Koike, T., Ohyama, K., Kawase, T., & Stephens, D. (2003). Transient evoked otoacoustic emissions in patients with middle ear disorders. *International Journal of Audiology, 42,* 117–131.

Index